the

CANCER
REVOLUTION

This book is dedicated to all of the people around the world who have or will face the challenges of cancer and believe that there are solutions and hope for the future.

the
CANCER
REVOLUTION

A Groundbreaking Program
to Reverse and Prevent Cancer

Leigh Erin Connealy, MD

Da Capo
LIFE
LONG

Set in 11 point Adobe Garamond Pro

Cataloging-in-Publication data for this book is available from the Library of Congress.

First Da Capo Press edition 2017

ISBN: 978-0-7382-1845-8 (hardcover)
ISBN: 978-0-7382-1846-5 (e-book)

Published by Da Capo Press, an imprint of Perseus Books, LLC, a subsidiary of Hachette Book Group, Inc.

www.dacapopress.com

Publisher's Note and Disclaimer: The opinions, views, and ideas in this book are solely those of the author and not of the publisher. The publisher does not endorse any such opinions, view or ideas, and cannot independently verify, and has not verified, the accuracy of the information contained in this book. This book is not intended to provide medical advice and should not be used as a basis to diagnose or treat any medical condition. For diagnosis or treatment of any medical problem, consult your own physician. This book is not intended to replace, contradict, supplant, countermand, or conflict with advice given to you by your own physician. References to sources provided in this book are informational only and do not constitute endorsement or sponsorship by the publisher of any such sources. Publisher disclaims all liability in connection with this book or any content it contains, or any reliance by you on that content.

Author's Disclaimer: The information in this book is not to be used to treat or diagnose any particular disease or particular patient. Neither the author nor the publisher is engaged in rendering professional advice or services to the individual reader. The ideas and recommendations in this book are not intended as a substitute for professional health care advice or a consultation with a professional health care provider. The publisher and authors are not responsible or liable for any adverse effects, losses, damages, or other consequences arising from any information or recommendations in this book. All matters pertaining to your personal health should be supervised by a healthcare professional.

Da Capo Press books are available at special discounts for bulk purchases in the U.S. by corporations, institutions, and other organizations. For more information, please contact the Special Markets Department at Perseus Books, 2300 Chestnut Street, Suite 200, Philadelphia, PA 19103, or call (800) 810-4145, ext. 5000, or e-mail special.markets @perseusbooks.com.

LSC-C

10 9 8 7 6 5

Contents

Foreword

Imagine a commercial plane crashed and people were killed. You can be sure that would make the headline of every major newspaper. Well, we have the equivalent of eight to ten planes crashing EVERY DAY with everyone onboard, dying from cancer.

Nearly 2 million Americans are diagnosed with cancer every year—one person out of three will be hit with a cancer diagnosis at some time in their lives, in spite of the massive technological advances over the past half-century. Western medicine is no closer to finding a "cancer cure," while cancer has grown into a worldwide epidemic of staggering proportions.

According to the CDC, about 1,660,290 (1.66 million) new cancer cases were diagnosed in 2014. Unfortunately, the cancer industry does not focus on effective *prevention* strategies, such as dietary guidelines, exercise, and obesity education. Instead, it pours its money into *treating cancer*, rather than preventing or curing it.

In spite of the enormous amounts of money funneled into cancer research today, two out of three cancer patients will be dead within five years after receiving all or part of the standard cancer treatment trinity—surgery, radiotherapy, and chemotherapy. This is not too surprising when you consider that two of the three traditional treatments are carcinogenic themselves! One study estimated that chemotherapy benefits about one of every twenty people receiving it.

Over the last hundred years, a number of natural cancer treatments have been developed and used successfully to treat patients in the United States and other countries. Most of these have been vehemently discounted, pushed under the rug by the medical monopoly, with physicians and researchers attacked, smeared, sent to prison, and professionally ruined for daring to defy the medical establishment—all to protect the financial interests of the pharmaceutical and medical industries. Drug companies have no interest in natural agents that they cannot patent, because they interfere with their revenue stream. They will go—and have gone—to extreme measures to prevent the truth about effective natural treatments from reaching the public.

Fortunately, you can learn about many cutting-edge cancer therapies by reading this book. Dr. Connealy carefully and clearly details the wide array of comprehensive strategies that you can consider for treating cancer. There really are an astounding number of choices and she does a magnificent job of compiling them conveniently in one place. It would take you many weeks, and more likely months or years, to collect the options that she concisely reviews here.

Not only does she outline the natural options for treating cancer, but she provides resources that you can use to identify a natural clinician that resonates with your philosophy and budget.

The Cancer Revolution will help you navigate the not widely publicized and frequently difficult to learn about alternatives that leading clinicians from around the world have been using to help put cancer into remission. It could save your life.

Dr. Joseph Mercola
Founder, Mercola.com, most-visited
natural health site on the Internet

PART ONE

A NEW WAY TO PREVENT,
TREAT, AND BEAT CANCER

CHAPTER 1

Cancer: What It Is, What Causes It, and How to Fight It

> **IN THIS CHAPTER, YOU WILL LEARN . . .**
>
> - Why cancer is a disease of the entire body, not a body part, and what tools you can use to help overcome it
> - How tumors are formed
> - Why the conventional approach isn't enough
> - Three main causes of cancer

One out of three women and one out of two men in the United States are developing cancer today. Most of us have lost a family member, a friend, or a colleague to cancer, or we know someone who has. Cancer is rampant: The National Institutes of Health has spent over a trillion dollars trying to find a cure, and yet the death rate from cancer is the same as what it was fifty years ago. For instance, one meta-analysis study by three Australian oncologists, the results of which were published in 2004 in the *Journal of Clinical Oncology*, revealed that the five-year survival rate for cancer of all types and stages is only about 60 percent, and that chemotherapy increases that five-year survival rate by only about 2 percent.[1] Further, conventional cancer treatments, while sometimes useful and necessary, may have the potential to harm some patients just as much as, if not more than, the cancer itself.

Early on in my career, I realized that chemotherapy, radiation, and surgery weren't enough to cure cancer, and my experience with thousands of patients over the years has solidified that belief. These treatments have their place in the fight against cancer, but by themselves they are inadequate, and when improperly used, can be dangerous. Also, cancer is a disease of the whole person, not a body part, yet most conventional oncologists treat cancer as a separate entity or as a specific problem in the body. They don't address the entire person or try to discover the root cause of disease; their aim is to kill the cancer rather than heal the body from the inside out. Instead of building up the immune system, which is the body's most effective and important weapon in the fight against cancer, conventional treatments tear it down and can sometimes create new health problems for the person.

Another reason the mainstream approach is inadequate is neither chemotherapy nor radiation nor surgery can eliminate what are called circulating tumor cells (CTCs) or cancer stem cells (CSCs). These are cells that break off from the original tumor and float around in the bloodstream (a process called metastasis), looking for their next "nest." CTCs and CSCs are responsible for more than 95 percent of all metastases and cancer deaths, but scientists haven't figured out a perfect, surefire way to eradicate them, so conventional treatments fall short on this crucial front. Further, these treatments don't address any of the cancer's survival mechanisms or the body's functional imbalances. Cancer is caused by the deregulation of multiple genes, which must be individually targeted by different natural anticancer agents.

Another major con of conventional treatments is they leave patients with a weakened immune system, which in turn increases their risk of cancer reoccurrence, contracting other illnesses, or suffering complications after surgery. Meanwhile, they live in the shadow of a ruthless disease that could return at any time.

Increasingly, cancer patients are also discovering that conventional care, with its five- or six-figure price tag, is not doing what it is supposed to. Many people have survived chemotherapy, radiation, and surgery, only to relapse and have to endure the process all over again. Despite these problems with conventional care, we keep doing the same thing over and over again, and getting the same results. This is the definition of insanity!

Fortunately, I have learned many things about cancer and cancer treatment that I think will encourage you. First, a cancer diagnosis does not have to be a death sentence. Science has provided us with new, cutting-edge tools that not only can accurately detect the disease better than before and earlier on, but which can also help you manage it so that you can live longer and experience a better quality of life.

Second, there are groundbreaking new cancer treatments in integrative medicine that are gentler than what's found in conventional medicine, and which are unlikely to cause terrible side effects, such as vomiting, hair loss, and fatigue. These treatments are useful, no matter what stage or type of cancer you have, and some can be used even if you just want to prevent cancer.

Finally, research suggests that such factors as diet, detoxification, exercise, nutritional supplements, stress management, sleep, and resolving emotional conflicts can, in some cases, trump any genetic predisposition to cancer. This means that your destiny doesn't have to be determined by your genes. If you understand this, then you can have a greater likelihood of being victorious over cancer and your health.

In *The Cancer Revolution*, I will empower you with an amazing arsenal of tools that can help you manage and fight cancer or prevent it from happening in the first place.

We encourage you to keep an open mind, as these tools and treatments aren't based on fads or some random philosophy. Instead, they are supported by many doctors' experiences with their patients, and I personally have witnessed some of my patients live long, productive lives as a result of doing them—not to mention the thousands of Pubmed articles on these topics. You probably won't hear about them in mainstream medicine, though, because most oncologists have only been taught to give their patients drugs, and so they don't understand or know about integrative methods. Also, integrative, homeopathic, and conventional Western medicines are not marketed to the same degree. Since many integrative natural therapies are not FDA approved, they are not advertised as prominently, which means they remain relatively unknown.

Yet integrative medicine is truly beneficial because it marries the best of conventional medicine with new, natural medicine, and is based on the idea that you must treat the root cause of disease, not just the tumor or cancer, and heal the *entire* person. This approach can produce exceptional outcomes.

Integrative medicine can include treatments from a wide variety of medical disciplines including homeopathic, nutritional, bioenergetic, regenerative, antiaging, and Chinese herbal medicine, along with lifestyle approaches to wellness.

Time and again, doctors who practice integrative medicine have found ways to help leverage the effects of conventional treatments, helping even the sickest of people strengthen their armor against cancer. And as our "best of both worlds" methods have made waves, these clinics have earned a reputation for being compassionate as well as patient because it is time to get to the root of our patients' problems.

As I mentioned, chemotherapy, radiation, and surgery do have their place in cancer treatment, but they are not enough, because regardless of the healing approach you decide to take—whether conventional or integrative—you *still* need to support your body before, during, and after cancer treatment. That means doing things like providing it with the nutrition it needs; detoxifying it from environmental pollutants; and protecting it against some of the harmful effects that chemotherapy, radiation, and other harsh treatments unfortunately can impose. It also means addressing all of the cancer's survival mechanisms, as well as all of your body's functional imbalances, which conventional treatment alone cannot do.

For instance, you might have low thyroid function, or inflammation, or high blood sugar, or a liver detoxification problem—all of which you would need to treat, along with the cancer, if you wanted to be well. You need to change your internal environment so that it becomes an inhospitable place for the cancer and it has a harder time surviving in your body.

In this book, I will teach you how to do all of these things. Even if conventional treatments alone have failed you, the approaches I will discuss have the potential to help you live a better quality of life. In my personal experience, I have seen many late-stage cancer patients who were told by their oncologists that they had only months or weeks left to live survive longer than their original prognoses. Even if you have a so-called deadly cancer, such as melanoma or pancreatic cancer, you will find tools and treatments in *The Cancer Revolution* that can help you improve your health and enjoy a better quality of life than you might have otherwise had. But you must first understand a few key things about cancer, including:

- How it develops in your body and what you can do to interfere with that process
- How to make lifestyle choices every day that can reduce your cancer risk
- How to use research to help support a loved one who has been diagnosed with cancer

Notice that my focus here has not been on how genetics factor into cancer risk and recovery. Many of us have been taught that if one of our close family members has or had cancer, then we're doomed to get cancer by default. But this is simply not true for every individual. The emerging science of epigenetics suggests that our genes are not our destiny. In fact, genes only contribute to 5 percent or less of our cancer risk (according to the American Cancer Society, "only about 5% to 10% of all cancers result directly from gene mutations that are inherited from a parent").[2] Even so, we can change how our genes are expressed by modifying our lifestyle, such as our dietary and exercise habits; by managing our stress levels, and detoxifying our body from environmental pollutants—just to name a few things. Many of the factors that activate cancer-causing genes and initiate the development of cancer are within your ability to prevent. In *The Cancer Revolution,* I will show you exactly how to do that.

Cancer: An Earthquake in Your Body

I like to tell my patients that cancer is an uncontrollable growth of cells in the body that have gone wild and crazy because they are overwhelmed or overstressed. These cells have been damaged by carcinogens, or cancer-causing toxins, which cause them to mutate and behave abnormally. Once they do this, they then become like an earthquake in the body and everything in it then gets thrown into chaos. It then takes years and a whole team of people and machines to rebuild and repair the damage.

Similarly, once you get cancer, you need a whole team of doctors and treatments to create order and restore homeostasis, or balance, to your body. And that repair isn't done in a month, or three, or six; it takes time. But if you understand this, you can then learn about what you need to do to heal yourself. We can actually make our patients feel a lot better in just a couple of weeks, by giving them such things as intravenous vitamin infusions, hyperbaric oxygen, and other therapies; by putting them on the right diet; and helping them spiritually. Yet the full healing and rebuilding process takes time—months or years, depending upon the damage that's been done.

You may find that your doctor can do things to help you feel better right away, but the process of repairing your body may take longer if only conventional methods are used. In Chapter 10, I will show you how to find a good integrative doctor and put together a healing team that can help you do this if you don't already have one.

Cancer is a disease of the *entire* body, not just a body part. A person doesn't just have breast, ovarian, or colon cancer, for instance, because the disease doesn't only affect the breasts, or the ovaries, or the colon—but the entire body, always and without exception. So, if you have a doctor that goes on the offensive and just attacks the tumor, or treats only the area of your body with cancer, then he or she is ignoring the fact that the cancer is a result of sickness in your entire body, and that it isn't just the tumor that needs to be treated, but *all of you*. Your "inner terrain" must be rebuilt and repaired, so that the root cause of disease can be removed.

What Causes Cancer?

Identifying the exact cause of cancer has proven tricky for scientists. After all, if we knew the cause, we'd be closer to finding a cure. However, a wealth of scientific research suggests a specific set of risk factors for the disease.

Today, practically everyone knows that smoking cigarettes is linked to an increased risk of developing lung cancer, but how many know that there are more than thirty different factors that can lead to cancer? They can be grouped into three basic categories: infections (bugs), toxins, and biological factors. All of these things may cause cancer by disrupting the body's homeostasis, research suggests.[3] One way they do this is by creating oxidative stress and inflammation. Inflammation and free radicals damage the RNA and DNA (the genetic material) inside the cells, and with that, the cells' mitochondria, or energy-producing furnaces.

When the mitochondria are damaged and a cell can no longer efficiently produce energy for itself, it reverts to an inefficient method of energy production called glycolysis, in which it depends on sugar as a fuel source. In this state, the organs and body systems can no longer work properly. This leads to more DNA damage, less energy for normal cells, and more fuel for cancer cells.

Environmental Toxins

Environmental toxins are one of the biggest causes of DNA damage and cellular mutations. The following is a list of some toxins that research links to cancer. I have divided them into two categories. The first describes toxins you are probably aware of and which you may already know can cause cancer. The second describes toxins that you may have heard of, but which you may not know are associated with cancer. In Chapter 5, I will share with you how you can help eliminate these toxins from your body and environment.

The "Usual" Suspects

- **Tobacco and smoking**
- **Mercury toxicity**—This comes from contaminated fish, water, air, and amalgam dental fillings (among other sources).
- **Sunlight**—The shortwave rays of the sun cause reddening and sunburn and damage the superficial epidermal layers of the skin.

Other Toxins

- **Electromagnetic fields**—Excessive exposure to electromagnetic fields (from microwave towers, cell phones, Wi-Fi, etc.) can cause cellular mutations that may lead to cancer.
- **Geopathic stress**—This comes from energies with the Earth that are created by underground cavitations, streams, and other geological features. Such energies are harmful to the body.[4]
- **Food additives**—These are substances added to food to preserve its flavor or enhance its taste and appearance. They include things such as stabilizers, food coloring, dyes, and artificial sweeteners.
- **Foci infections, especially dental infections**—Many of us have hidden foci infections in the body, which are concentrated and localized pockets of infection that don't show up on routine lab tests. Among the most insidious and damaging of these are infections that are found in the mouth, and which are produced by root canals and jawbone infections. These infections produce toxins that could lead to inflammation and cancer.[5]
- **Immunosuppressives and other drugs**
- **Industrial toxins**—These are ubiquitous in our air, food, and water supply. Industrial toxins, such as ammonia, fluoride, and chlorine, can be found in recycled water/tap water. For a list of all the common environmental toxins, go to the United States Department of Labor website: https://www.osha.gov/SLTC/emergency preparedness/guides/chemical.html.

- **Ionizing radiation**—This comes from such tests as X-rays and CT scans. Radiation can increase an individual's cancer risk.[6]
- **Irradiated food**—Some of our food supply, especially spices, fruits, and meat, is irradiated to eliminate organisms that cause foodborne illness and to preserve the shelf life of food. This radiation damages the body. Although irradiated foods are common and found almost everywhere, there are clear ways to avoid them, such as buying produce from farmers' markets, asking whether your produce contain GMOs, and growing your own fruits and vegetables.
- **Nuclear radiation**—This comes from power plant accidents, such as what happened at the Fukushima power plant in 2011 in Japan.
- **Pesticides**—These are sprayed on fruits and vegetables to keep pathogens from destroying them.
- **Polluted water**—Tap water may contain such things as chlorine, fluorine, pharmaceutical drugs, parasites and other microbes, and other chemicals linked to cancer.
- **"Sick building" syndrome**—This is caused by buildings that are contaminated by mold and other biotoxins.
- **Xenoestrogens**—These come from plastics and other chemical compounds that mimic the effects of human estrogen upon the body.

As you can see, there are many more environmental toxins and factors that are linked to cancer than what you may have been aware of!

Infections: Viruses, Bacteria, Parasites, and Fungi

Viruses, bacteria, parasites, and fungi, such as molds, mildews, and *Candida*, cause inflammation in the body and can increase cancer risk.

Certain infections have also been directly linked to specific types of cancer. For instance, the human papilloma virus (HPV) has been associated with head and neck cancers, as well as cervical cancer. Epstein-Barr virus (EBV) is associated with leukemia. Hepatitis C has been linked to liver cancer, and colitis is related to colon cancer. Herpes II increases cancer risk in general.

You may not always know whether you have an infection in your body that's creating an environment that is favorable to the development of cancer. A good integrative doctor can help you identify and eliminate any low-grade or underlying acute and chronic infections. Treating infections can help lower your risk of any cancers that may be directly caused by those infections.

Biological Factors

Other factors that may cause cancer include:

- **A poor diet and nutritional deficiencies**—Much of our soil is nutrient-depleted and loaded with pesticides and other toxins, as are some of the foods that line our supermarket shelves. Also, many people don't consume whole foods and instead opt for processed, unhealthy, nutrient-depleted food.
- **Toxic emotions and chronic stress**—We describe stress and emotions in greater detail later in this book. Experimental studies have shown that stress can affect a tumor's ability to grow and spread.[7]
- **Depressed thyroid function**—This can result from gluten allergies, heavy metal toxins, radiation exposure, fluoride consumption, iodine deficiencies, and autoimmune disease, among other factors.
- **Intestinal toxicity**—Many of us have an unhealthy gastrointestinal tract due to infections or because we eat harmful foods. Antibiotics, pesticides, and other environmental contaminants, as well as pathogenic infections and other factors, damage beneficial bacteria and the mucosa of the stomach and intestines.
- **Unbalanced "cellular terrain"**—The internal terrain of your body determines how well every cell is oxygenated and nourished. Pathogens grow in the body when its internal terrain is out of balance. Nutritional imbalances, toxins, and acidic waste also contribute to an unhealthy terrain.
- **Hormone therapies**—Birth control pills, synthetic estrogen hormone replacement therapy, and hormone blockers disrupt the body's hormones and cause biochemical imbalances that may lead to cancer. RBSt, a synthetic hormone given to cows to accelerate their growth and that is found in conventionally processed meat and dairy products, can also cause imbalances.
- **Compromised detoxification**—Your body's ability to remove toxins can be compromised by bad circulation, scars, and other factors.

- **Cellular oxygen deficiency**—This is caused by excessive acidity in the body, as well as by a lack of exercise, pollution, and/or a lack of carbon dioxide in the cells.

According to American Medical Research LLC (AMR), a medical research company, toxins are responsible for 70 to 75 percent of all cancers. Viruses and other infections cause 20 to 25 percent of all cancers, and electromagnetic pollution and genetics are thought to cause less than 5 percent each of all cancers.[8]

Otto Warburg, a Nobel Prize winner, German physician, and physiologist, discovered that cancer occurs when any cell is denied 60 percent of its oxygen.[9] Poor oxygenation results from a buildup of carcinogens and other toxins inside of and around the cells, which then damages the cell's ability to utilize oxygen. Additionally, psychological and emotional stress and nutritional imbalances are important contributing factors to cancer, although researchers aren't sure to what degree they play a role in its development. In *The Cancer Revolution*, I will show you how you can remove the effects of all of these factors from your body, so that you can either continue to live a cancer-free life, or help fight a cancer you may already have.

Finally, the following are some additional facts about cancer that you may not know:

- Some studies link sugar to the growth of cancer cells. Sugar may increase the risk of certain types of cancer.[10]
- A sedentary lifestyle creates a lack of oxygen in the body and can contribute to cancer growth.
- Bacteria, viruses, toxins, parasites, and heavy metals may indirectly increase cancer growth by suppressing the immune system.
- You are more likely to get cancer if your immune system is already compromised. According to the Canadian Cancer Society, a compromised immune system increases an individual's chances of contracting different viruses and bacteria that can increase the risk of cancer.

How Tumors Are Formed

Every cell has the capacity to become a cancer cell under the right conditions. When a normal cell becomes damaged and mutates, it ceases to work as part of the team and community of other cells that it is a part of, and instead starts to work for itself, for its own survival. As part of this process, it grows rapidly and doesn't respond to the body's natural cellular control mechanisms.

So, tumors start with a normal cell mutating into an "immortal," uncooperative cancer cell. This cell then multiplies and proliferates until it becomes a mass of cells. Once this mass reaches a certain level, it seeks to form a "nest" somewhere in the body, and by this means it begins to establish itself in a specific organ or set of tissues to become what we know as a tumor.

As the tumor grows larger, it begins to require greater and greater amounts of nutrients from the blood, until it finally creates its own set of blood vessels and blood supply in a process called angiogenesis. Finally, if left unchecked, some of the cancer cells will break off from the tumor and establish new tumors, or "nests," in other parts of the body (metastasis).

Normally, your immune system will detect and destroy any cancer cells before they are able to form a colony of cells or a tumor. But if your immune system is compromised by toxins or infections, and is "blinded" by inflammation, cancer cells can more easily reproduce. As the cancer cells reproduce, they coat themselves with a substance called fibrin, which helps them hide from the immune system and stick together and form a colony. That colony will then attach to a wall in your smooth muscle and begin developing blood vessels so that it can get more nutrients from your blood to feed itself.

To further enable its survival, the newly developed tumor will send out a lot of other information, in signals known as growth factors, to the rest of the body that will aid in its growth and development. There are many different signals that tumors put out, so it's important to prevent or halt these transmissions. Cancer has multiple survival strategies, all of which need to be addressed with different treatments, at the same time that your body must be repaired and restored from the "earthquake."

Can We Prevent Cancer?

Although many factors in our environment cause cancer, and cancer has multiple survival mechanisms to help it grow in the body, most of the time we *can* prevent it! According to a recent Japanese study, we all have 75 million cancer cells in our body at any given time.[11] Normally, our immune system keeps these cells in check, but when the immune system becomes compromised over a long period of time, these cells can begin to proliferate, or multiply. But we can help stop this process by consuming a nutritious diet.

It takes ten to twelve years on average for a single cancer cell to eventually multiply to where it becomes a full-grown tumor in the body. This means you often have a lot of time to eliminate the things that are causing cancer, if you catch it in the early stages. There are early-detection tests that you can do, such as the Cancer Profile, which I describe in greater detail in Chapter 2. This test, among others, aims to help determine whether the environment in your body is favorable to the development of cancer, or whether cancer is already "brewing or fermenting" somewhere in it, many years before it actually becomes a disease.

Currently, not many doctors in the United States know how to *prevent* cancer because most are trained to be reactive with their patients instead of proactive. The good news is that increasingly, doctors are being trained in functional and integrative medicine and are helping their patients help prevent cancer, just as we do at our clinic. Cancer is a global illness, affecting the entire body; it's not just a disease of a single body part, so it's essential that you work with a doctor who can look at your entire body and tell you whether you have an internal environment that is favorable to its development. In Chapter 10 and the Resources section at the end of this book, I provide a list of referral organizations and tips that will help you find such a doctor.

To prevent or fight cancer, you must also resolve the stress and emotional conflicts in your life. I describe both of these factors in greater detail in Chapter 8. I often ask my patients whether they want to be well, and tell them, "I can't help you until you get your mind in order." You must want to be well and discipline yourself to do all the right things if you want to heal.

It's like weight loss. Unfortunately, according to the United Institute of Health and Human Services, about two thirds (68.8%) of the population is characterized as being overweight.[12] Some are overweight because they don't "pay attention to their intention" (their mind and thoughts). Everyone wants to pop a pill for every ill, but we have known for a long time that this doesn't work. So, why are we still looking to "pop a pill," when we know that doesn't work?

I sometimes tell our patients, "Do you know that very talented artists, musicians, and performers such as the most famous pianists in the world, even though they were born gifted, still have to practice the piano for five hours a day? Or, take famous basketball players, such as Kobe Bryant: Although he was born with the necessary height and talent to succeed in basketball, he still has to practice playing the sport daily. So it is with your health. You have to practice at being healthy because health is a process, not a one-time event. You don't just become healthy one day."

My daughter once said to me, "Mom, you are just so disciplined about the way you live." And I told her, "I have worked at my health my entire life, because I've faced great adversity. If I don't work at my health and if I'm not disciplined, then I pay for it. And I don't want to pay. I'd rather be disciplined and have a good outcome."

Another analogy I give my patients has to do with driving. I will say to them, "Do you drive? If you do, then you know that there is a rulebook for driving, and that you have to know the rules and laws of driving a car." Then I will ask them, "How many stop signs did you run today? None, right? Because you know that you'd probably get a ticket, hurt somebody, or crash the car if you did.

"Similarly, you have to pay attention to the rules of your body. Because nobody wants to get into a car accident, and I don't want you to have a body accident! If you follow the rules and laws of Mother Nature, then the right things will happen in your body."

It's not about perfection, though, because none of us are perfect drivers, and you aren't going to be a perfect driver with your health. But you want to follow the rules of nature so that your body works for you, not against you. What percentage of the time do you think you can get away with running a stop sign? Once in a while, right? But that's about it.

Preventing cancer doesn't need to be complicated. You just need to learn a few key things about how to be well, which you can do without spending a fortune. Likewise, if you have already been diagnosed with cancer, there are many simple lifestyle and dietary changes that you can make that can help you battle the disease and live a longer, more vibrant life, which you will find throughout this book.

JACK H's Story

In early 2013, I had a slight irritation at the back of my throat, which, after much testing, I discovered was squamous cell carcinoma. I don't have empirical proof, but I strongly suspect that the cancer was triggered by mold toxicity. My family and I were living in a house that was inundated with mold in the TV room and bedroom. We all have cancer cells in our body, but it was the mold in this house that I believe knocked down my immune system so that the cancer could run wild and multiply. My entire family had constant coughing, respiratory illnesses, and colds while living in that house.

After my diagnosis, my wife and I began researching cancer treatment options, including chemotherapy and radiation. I saw both integrative and traditional doctors, including a couple of doctors at a well-known university hospital (but I did not do chemotherapy or radiation with them). Now if you were to ask me about what I think of this hospital, I'd say that what they do mechanically, such as operating on the throat to remove a tumor, is terrific; they are as good as you can get! But when it comes to preventive care, they aren't even in the ballpark.

I told the doctors at the university, "You know, you want to do an MRI on me to look for cancer, but the MRI won't tell you anything about what's going on in my body, except that I have something there." And the MRI tells me nothing about how I can prevent getting cancer in the first place.

I concluded from my research and experience that a good definition for the kind of treatment that people with cancer should be getting is called "integrative medicine," which involves addressing not only the tumor but also things like your diet and lifestyle, and toxins like heavy metals and mold.

So, I chose to do integrative treatments with Dr. Connealy, who routinely does lots of blood tests to check the status of my health and make sure that something dangerous isn't developing in my body or hindering my recovery. The doctors at the university hospital did only one blood test on me, which was a pre-op blood test, and they didn't discuss the importance of a healthy diet or things that people with cancer should avoid, like sugar and excessively high amounts of carbohydrates.

I have never been afraid of cancer. When I got the diagnosis, it wasn't a death sentence to me, although other people I'd known who had cancer had seen it as such. But throughout my whole experience with it, I have never been afraid of it because I have always been in good shape and have kept myself in good condition. I have also found some great tools in integrative medicine that have been effective for fighting it. So, I never doubted that my body could take care of it, and today, I am doing well.

CHAPTER 2

How to Detect Cancer Before It Wreaks Havoc

IN THIS CHAPTER, YOU WILL LEARN . . .

- The top early-prevention screening tests
- How to increase your chances of detecting cancer before conventional tests
- The best treatments for your body and how to track your progress with them
- Symptoms that may indicate you have cancer

Whether you develop active cancer depends a lot upon you and the lifestyle and dietary choices that you make, which means that being healthy and cancer-free is largely within your control. You *can* help prevent cancer by eliminating from your body the toxins that cause it, eating the right foods, correcting nutritional imbalances, reducing emotional stress, and doing other things that I describe throughout *The Cancer Revolution*.

Just as important, you can find out whether cancer is "brewing" or "simmering" somewhere in your body, or whether you are likely to get it, by regularly doing cancer prevention screening tests. Contrary to popular belief, you can often detect cancer in its earliest stages, before it takes a noticeable toll on your health. This is because, as a general rule, and as I mentioned in Chapter 1, it takes an average of ten to twelve years for cancer to fully develop in the body, and eight years for a tumor to form. That means it's possible to get a jump start on halting its progression. In this chapter I will share some useful screening tools that can help you do this, so that you can help reduce your risk for developing cancer, and/or stop a potential cancer from taking over your body.

If you are reading this book because you have already been diagnosed with cancer, there is still a lot you can do to stop its progression and reverse it. This chapter outlines some useful diagnostic tests that will not only help you determine how far advanced the cancer is, but also what treatments would be most beneficial for you *personally*, and how you can get a decent idea of when the cancer is in remission.

You may find yourself overwhelmed with the amount of information that is presented here, and wonder how, what, and when you should do the different tests here described. Rather than decide by yourself what you need, I recommend reviewing and sharing this information with a skilled and experienced integrative doctor and certainly your primary oncologist, who can help you to determine which of the following tests you should do. Integrative doctors are likely to be familiar with some, if not most or all of these tests, unlike your conventional oncologist, who may or may not be familiar with them or willing to explore using them with you. However, being transparent with your regular oncologist is crucial for helping maximize the effectiveness of your cancer treatment and avoid potentially compromising your health.

If you don't already have a relationship with an integrative oncologist or holistic cancer doctor, you can find one in your area by doing a physician search at any one of the following medical association websites, which maintain a database of integrative cancer doctors:

- Academy for Comprehensive Integrative Medicine: www.acim connect.com
- American College for Advancement in Medicine: www.acam.org
- International Organization of Integrative Cancer Physicians: www .ioicp.com
- Best Answer for Cancer: www.bestanswerforcancer.org

In Chapter 10, I share some additional tips and strategies that will help you in your search for an integrative cancer doctor, along with how to put together an effective support system.

Another reason you should work with a skilled and experienced integrative doctor is this type of doctor will do a whole-body evaluation on you and not just treat the tumor, as may some conventional oncologists. Good integrative doctors conduct extensive blood tests to evaluate a wide variety of markers: those that relate directly to the cancer, as well as those that indirectly relate, such as your body's hormonal function. For instance, I have observed that if a patient is not producing adrenal hormones and his or her adrenal glands are weak, then we know that we need to support those glands; otherwise, his or her body won't be able to handle the cancer treatments very well. The doctor you choose to help you needs to know the overall functional status of your body. This is because, for example, if you are diabetic or have blood sugar regulation problems, low thyroid function, or high inflammatory markers, these medical conditions will impact your recovery. You want to make sure that your body is stable and that everything is in working order so your immune system can effectively fight the cancer, and most skilled integrative oncologists will understand this. A successful integrative cancer doctor will also know how to tailor a treatment plan to your specific needs. That personalization is key because every individual is an original and no two people require exactly the same plan.

The following are some excellent cancer prevention and screening tests that you will want to share with your doctor should you try them. These tests will tell you such things as whether you have cancer; how far advanced it is, and whether your current treatments are working. Again, the specific tests you'll want to do depends first and foremost upon whether you have cancer or are trying to prevent it, as well as the type and progression of the cancer. Most of these tests require a prescription from your doctor, which is another good reason to work with an integrative doctor who can help you to decide which ones you'll need to do.

Cancer Prevention and Screening Tests

The Cancer Profile

The Cancer Profile is a test that was developed by Emil Schandl, PhD, founder of American Metabolic Laboratories and Metabolic Research, Inc. Many integrative doctors recommend this preventive test to everyone because it enables you to identify cancer in its earliest developmental stages—as early as ten to twelve years before the tumor becomes detectable on other routine tests. The Cancer Profile provides early warning signs of cancer, but it can also be used to monitor established cancers, and help you and your doctor to determine whether your current treatment regimen is working, as well as what you might need to do to adjust it.

The Cancer Profile measures a wide range of markers in the body. One of the most important of these is HCG, which is a hormone that is normally produced during pregnancy, but which can also be a hormone of malignancy. Most cancers produce HCG, so if you have any amount of HCG in your blood, this could indicate a greater risk of cancer. The HCG test is a very simple blood test, and it checks for two subunits of HCG: two in the blood and one in the urine. Two tests are done to positively verify the diagnosis.

Another marker in the body that the Cancer Profile measures is an enzyme called PHI, or phosphohexose isomerase/glucose phosphate isomerase. PHI causes cells to change their metabolism to a process called glycolysis, in which cancer cells produce energy in a low-oxygen environment that enables their survival. If your PHI enzyme is elevated, then this means that your body is becoming a relatively more cancer-friendly environment.

According to Dr. Schandl, in an interview for the Alternative Cancer Research Institute,[1] if you have surgery to remove a tumor and your surgeon tells you the doctors have removed all the cancer cells, if your PHI enzyme tests are positive, then this is not true—you still have cancer. The tumor may be gone, but the cancer has likely already started establishing itself somewhere else in your body.

The Cancer Profile also measures your thyroid hormone function. Your thyroid is your body's "battery," and thyroid hormones are responsible for your body's basic metabolic rate, which is linked to the amount of oxygen your body uses and its availability to the tissues. The idea behind the test is the more oxygen your cells have, the fewer cancer cells you will have in your body.

In addition, the test measures a liver enzyme called gamma-glutamyltran-speptidase (GGTP), and nonspecific tumor markers called CEA and DHEA sulfate. The liver is your body's primary detoxification organ, and the GGTP is a great test that can suggest markers for liver disease or damage. GGTP levels are also increased in certain types of cancer, especially metastatic liver cancer, pancreatic carcinomas, and breast and colon cancers that have metas-tasized to the liver, so it can be a great cancer marker test as well. CEA is a broad-spectrum cancer antigen—that is, a protein foreign to the body that provokes an immune response—that can be found in some cases of cancer.

Finally, DHEA is an adrenal hormone that helps the body cope with stress, and which promotes longevity and proper immune function when levels are normal. According to Dr. Schandl, most people, if not everyone with cancer, has a very low DHEA level, which means that their immune system is suppressed. The Cancer Profile will indicate whether your DHEA level is low.

The Cancer Profile is a great tool that can help you to prevent cancer by showing you and your doctor what you might need to address to improve your health status, or it can help you check your progress on your current cancer treatment protocol. You don't need a prescription to order the Cancer Profile; however, I recommend working with a doctor, who can better help you interpret the results and formulate a treatment plan based on those results. To learn more and to order the test, see the Resources section at the end of this book.

ONCOblot

Another useful blood test for detecting cancer in the early stages is the ONCOblot. This is a new test that has only been available since January 2013 and that is able to detect over twenty-six known forms of cancer, seven to eight years before a tumor shows up on conventional scans. It can also show you in what organ(s) the cancer is developing. ONCOblot Labs is in the process of seeking FDA approval; the test currently meets FDA requirements for a Laboratory Developed Test (LDT).

The ONCOblot checks your body for a special kind of protein called ENOX2 that exists only on the surface of cancer cells. These proteins are shed into the circulation and can be detected in the blood, and serve as highly sensitive markers for the early detection of both primary and recurrent cancers.

The ONCOblot can detect a cancer mass that contains only 2 million cells. Compare this to a positive mammogram, which can only find cancer once the mass has reached 4.5 trillion cells. The ONCOblot test can only be ordered by a physician. To find one that does this type of testing, you can visit the ONCOblot website for a referral, or ask your doctor to order the test for you. For more information, see the Resources section at the end of this book.

Research Genetic Cancer Center

The two tests that I just described are great if you want to prevent cancer or find out if you already have a cancer developing somewhere in your body. But if you already know that you have cancer, there are additional tests that you and your doctor should do, and which we also recommend to our patients at the Center. These tests can help you determine such things as circulating tumor cells and circulating stem cells, as well as the kinds of chemo and natural treatments that have the best likelihood of working for you, and help you evaluate your progress on your current treatment regimen.

One of the reasons why the conventional approach to cancer often falls short is that surgery, chemotherapy, and radiation can't eliminate what are called circulating tumor cells (CTCs) or cancer stem cells (CSCs), which are responsible for 95 percent of all metastases and deaths from cancer. You can find out whether you have CTCs and CSCs in your blood, and how many, by doing a blood test through Research Genetic Cancer Center (RGCC), a laboratory in Greece that conducts blood tests to check for both CTCs and CSCs. RGCC was officially established in 2004 and has over ten years of experience in working with doctors worldwide.

If, for instance, you had surgery to remove the six inches of your colon that had cancer, the RGCC test would show whether you truly were cancer-free by checking for any remaining CTCs and CSCs that came from the original tumor. The most accurate way to help determine whether you have eradicated cancer is when your CTC and CSC levels are zero. Within the integrative medical community, it is widely accepted that tumors that become larger than 1 to 2 millimeters in size have cells that have likely broken off from them and migrated into the circulatory system. These cells are dangerous because they can eventually build a "nest" somewhere else in your body and create new tumors. So, it is important to eliminate CTCs as well as the original tumor.

Then there are cancer stem cells, which are found within a tumor and which also can't be eliminated with conventional therapy. They can self-renew and regrow the tumor, after the tumor has been shrunken by such treatments as chemotherapy.

If you find through the RGCC test that you have CTCs or CSCs, the good news is you can take steps to help eliminate them! This is because RGCC doesn't just test for the presence of these cells in your body, but also exposes them to forty-nine of the most commonly used natural anticancer agents, to see which ones they will best respond to. Therefore, unlike standardized therapy, RGCC will tell you what treatments are the most effective for the genetics and type of cancer that you have. Your doctor can then choose from among these agents to formulate a treatment plan for you.

Integrative oncologists use this type of testing to determine what cancer treatment agents our patients need, especially those who are receiving either low-dose chemotherapy (which is explained in Chapter 3) from us or full-dose chemotherapy from their oncologist, and who want to know what anticancer agents are best for them.

Like the ONCOblot test, the RGCC test can only be ordered by a doctor. Not all cancer doctors are aware of the RGCC test, but many experienced and knowledgeable integrative oncologists will be. You can find a list of doctors in the United States that do RGCC testing by going to the RGCC website for your particular country, and clicking on "Doctor Locator" on the top menu. So, for instance, to find a doctor in your state in the United States that does RGCC testing, you would go to: http://www.rgccusa.com /doctor-locator/. When researching integrative oncologists, you can also ask them whether they do this type of testing. The RGCC is one of the most important tests for determining exactly what treatments your particular cancer will respond to, so we highly recommend finding a doctor that uses it.

Thermography

Breast cancer is the most common type of cancer in the United States, with about 235,000 people, mostly women, diagnosed in 2014, according to the National Cancer Institute.[2] Typically, conventional doctors will recommend that after age fifty women do a yearly mammogram, which is an X-ray exam of the breast that's used to detect cancer. But unfortunately, mammography is not very accurate for diagnosing breast cancer. According to an article in *The Lancet*, of the 5 percent of mammograms that suggest further testing, as high as 93 percent show up as false positives.[3]

A lesser-known way to help find out whether you are at risk for breast cancer or already have it is through thermography testing. Thermography uses infrared imaging technology to detect and measure heat and vascular patterns within the breast that can indicate cancer. Thermography can also detect abnormal findings in the breast. It can also be used to track your progress on a treatment regimen, and is safe, noncontact, and pain- and radiation-free.

My colleague Martin Bales, LAc, PhD, a board-certified thermologist and licensed acupuncturist, uses a sophisticated thermography device to screen patients for breast cancer. The thermography device can track inflammatory processes, but more important, it reveals vascular or vein patterns in the breast. These patterns look a bit like "spider veins"—and can help measure an individual's cancer risk. The more extensive the vein patterns, the more likely it is that a woman is either at risk for cancer or already has cancer, and it is thought to be especially so if the breasts are asymmetrical, and when one breast has more vein development than the other. The veins may suggest that the body is creating new blood vessels to feed a tumor. The website Mypinkimage.com shows some examples of these vascular patterns.

It is normal to have veins in your body, around the areas of your extremities (e.g., wrists), but you aren't supposed to have a lot of veins in your breasts. Of course, these veins are only visible on a thermography device, not visually, but if they show up on the device, then this means that there is a possibility that cancer could be brewing in your body. Dr. Bales says that in younger women, these veins are linked primarily to the use of birth control pills, and in older women, by the use of synthetic hormone replacement therapy (HRT). The other main associations with these veins are soy and flaxseed. Many people nowadays know that soy isn't a perfect health food, but most people still think that flax is harmless. Soy and flaxseed contain phytoestrogens, which are thought to mimic the effects of natural estrogen upon the body.[4] Many people today are estrogen-dominant; meaning they have too much estrogen, and this can contribute to the development of some types of reproductive cancers, such as breast cancer. Dr. Bales contends that when women quit taking birth control and HRT therapy, and stop consuming flax and soy, their vascular patterns often change for the better.

One thing that's important to understand about thermography is the color and heat pattern function of the thermography device doesn't reveal whether you have breast cancer, yet many practitioners use the heat pattern function of the device to scan their patients for breast cancer. So, I believe it is beneficial to find a technician or doctor who understands the importance of looking at vascular patterns in your breast, not just areas of inflammation in your body. You can find a competent technician or doctor in your area that looks at vascular breast patterns by asking for a referral at the International Academy of Clinical Thermology, or by researching physicians at one of the medical association databases listed earlier in this chapter. See the Resources for more information.

Thermography can also be useful for revealing the amount of xenoestrogens ("foreign estrogens," as translated from the original Greek) and phytoestrogens that are in your body. Xenoestrogens are chemicals that come from environmental toxins and are a primary cause of cancer. If you find that you have an abnormal vein pattern, you may want to ask your doctor to do a test through Genova Diagnostic Laboratories to find out how many xen-oestrogenic toxins, including phthalates and parabens, you have in your body. These chemicals may disrupt hormones, particularly estrogen, by binding to your body's estrogen receptors. They have the potential to trigger abnormal vein patterns in the breast, so you'll want to find out whether you have these kinds of toxins in your body, and if so, get them removed. In Chapter 5, I'll show you how to do that.

I Sensitivity C-Reactive Protein

This simple blood test is a nonspecific marker for inflammation, which is a precursor to all chronic, degenerative diseases, such as Alzheimer's, heart disease, and cancer. If you have elevated and ongoing levels of C-reactive protein (CRP), I'd advise your doctor to conduct a diagnostic test for cancer. CRP is a routine test that you can order from online laboratory services, such as Direct Labs (see Resources), without a prescription and then do it yourself at your local lab. However, as with all of the tests mentioned in this chapter, it's best to work with an integrative doctor—along with your current oncologist—who can determine what your body most needs based on your test results.

Hemoglobin A1c (HbA1c)

This is another simple test you can order without a prescription that measures your average blood sugar level over the past three months. It's important that you know what your HbA1c is because some studies suggest sugar may increase the risk of certain types of cancer, as well as diabetes and obesity, which can further contribute to this chance, according to the Mayo Clinic. As a precaution, I would recommend following a low-sugar and low-carb diet. In Chapter 4, we describe an ideal low-carb diet for cancer patients.

Bioenergetic Testing

Bioenergetic testing is a great complement to blood and other types of testing. It utilizes the energy of your body, along with a computerized device, to scan your body. Bioenergetic testing can tell you such things as what toxins and infections you have, as well as how well your hormones, glands, and organs are functioning. It can also help your doctor determine whether you have an environment in your body that may be more favorable to the development of cancer, and help him or her prioritize your health issues, and decide which ones need to be treated first.

Bioenergetic testing can also help determine the specific remedies or treatments that are most likely to benefit you. I know from clinical experience what my patients are likely to need, but bioenergetic testing can tell me, for instance, the specific products, not just the type of product, that they need. For example, I recently checked a patient's adrenal gland function through bioenergetic testing, and the scan revealed that a Biotics product would be best for helping her adrenals heal. There is a vast array of adrenal products out there, not all of which would have benefited this patient, so the testing helped me to narrow down, from among the products, the one that was most likely to produce the best results for her.

One of the best bioenergetic devices that many integrative practitioners use is called the limbic stress assessment (LSA) system, which was created by the ZYTO Corporation. The LSA system is a computerized electrodermal screening device that measures the electrical resistance on the surface of your hands, and based on this resistance, detects energy imbalances in your body. The energy imbalances are meant to reveal what problems are going on in your body and where.

For this test, a communication link is established between you, the patient, and a computer via a hand cradle. Through this connection, the LSA sends stimuli to your body and then records your body's energetic response. This conversation between you and the device is called biocommunications, and it can offer insights to you and your doctor about the treatments that you are most likely to need. It can also help identify the particular nutritional supplements and foods that would most likely benefit you, and can even aid in uncovering infections you may have. For example, the printout that the LSA generates might show whether there are bacteria, viruses, or parasites in your body, and provide a listing of the specific supplements that will serve to eliminate those infections and restore your body to homeostasis, or balance.

Not all integrative doctors do this type of testing, but many do, and it is a great complement to the other tests described in this chapter. So, it is ideal, although not essential, to find a practitioner that does this type of testing, in addition to the other lab tests that I have described in this chapter. To find a doctor that uses the LSA, you can ask for a recommendation from the ZYTO Corporation (see the Resources section for contact information). You could also do an Internet search for a doctor who does bioenergetic testing in your area. Use the terms "bioenergetic testing" or "ZYTO" or "LSA testing," and then put the name of your city and state into the search box. There are other types of bioenergetic testing devices and methods that function similarly to the LSA test, but in my experience, I have found the LSA to be one of the most accurate, which is why I recommend it here. Increasingly, more doctors are doing bioenergetic testing in addition to blood, urine, stool, and saliva tests, so with a little persistence, you are likely to find one that incorporates this kind of testing into his or her overall evaluation.

Meridian Stress Assessment Testing

The Chinese discovered thousands of years ago that we all have measurable energy channels in our bodies that correlate with and which are connected to specific organs and systems. Then, in the 1940s, a German medical doctor and engineer named Reinhard Voll started using instruments to measure the electrical conductance along these channels, and through his testing, he discovered areas of concentrated energy that we now refer to as acupuncture points. He then created a computerized device that could measure the health of the organs based on the energy of the pathways and the acupuncture points to which they are connected. Any disruption or abnormality in any of the pathways meant that there was a problem in an organ or tissue along that particular pathway. From his discoveries, meridian stress assessment testing was developed.

Meridian stress assessment testing, another bioenergetic diagnostic tool that many integrative doctors use, uses the acupuncture points on the patient's fingers and toes to determine how energy is flowing throughout different channels of the body.

BioMeridian devices can detect specific remedies that will bring your body back into energetic balance. Just as important, BioMeridian testing aims to identify where the cancer is in your body, and reveal how far along you are in the twelve-year cancer development process, which we call the "Cancer Cascade." Knowing what point you are at in the "Cascade" can help you and your doctor determine the aggressiveness of your treatment. It is a very reliable, valuable cancer detection test. To find a practitioner in your area, consult the Alternatives for Healing medical directory website (see the Resources section) or do a search by typing the term "BioMeridian practitioner" into the website search box, along with your city and state. So, for example, if you live in Los Angeles, you would type "BioMeridian practitioner, Los Angeles, California" into the search box.

PET and CT Scans, MRIs, X-rays, and Ultrasound Tests

Other cancer screening tests that integrative doctors may also incorporate in their evaluation processes include the positron emission tomography (PET) scan, computed tomography (CT) scan, magnetic resonance imaging (MRI), chest X-ray, and ultrasound. These are more traditional tests that are also commonly used by conventional oncologists.

A PET scan uses radiation to produce three-dimensional, color images of the functional processes within your body. PET scans can reveal where the cancer is, as well as the extent of the illness. But for the test to be useful, the cancer has to have reached a size that is large enough for it to be detected on the scan because you can have cancer yet have a normal PET scan. So, a certain volume of cancer cells must be present for the cancer to show up on the scan. Also, you may have a large amount of circulating tumor cells that haven't yet "nested" anywhere in your body, and a PET scan will not be able to detect those, either.

We recommend this kind of test to our patients less frequently than we do some of the others mentioned in this chapter because the radiation from a PET scan is six hundred times that of a chest X-ray, and some studies suggest too much exposure to radiation can be harmful.

PET scans are helpful, though, in certain cases, such as when there's an obstruction in your body or something else of importance that requires immediate attention. PET scans are also helpful for determining the extent of disease. For instance, they can reveal whether the cancer is localized, or has spread to other parts of your body.

Other tests that skilled integrative and conventional doctors use include CT or MRI scans. MRIs use magnetism and radio waves to create computer-generated pictures of the soft tissue parts of your body that are sometimes hard to see using other imaging tests. This imaging can help find some types of cancers and can tell you and your doctor whether a tumor is benign or cancerous. MRIs do not expose the body to radiation.

X-rays and CT scans can also be useful for showing the shape, size, and location of a tumor. CT scans and X-rays are similar. The main difference is an X-ray test aims a broad beam of radiation at your body from only one angle, whereas a CT scan uses a thin beam to take pictures of the organs and soft tissues from different angles. While these tests are useful and at times necessary, they do emit radiation (although much less than that which comes from a PET scan).

Ultrasound testing is another common and popular tool for detecting some cancers. With it, doctors can also distinguish cysts from solid tumors because they create very different echo patterns.

If you have cancer or suspect that you have cancer, you don't need to worry about which of these tests you might need to do, as a competent integrative doctor in conjunction with your regular doctor will be able to determine that for you. We just share them here so that you have an idea about the wide variety of diagnostic tools that are available in integrative medicine and understand why it's important for your doctor to use multiple types of tests in your evaluation.

Other Cancer Screening Tests

Doctors of conventional medicine also utilize mammography, pap smears, and colonoscopy testing to screen for breast, cervical, and colon cancers, respectively. Unfortunately, these tests can only detect cancer once it has reached a certain size in the body, so their usefulness is limited.

Similarly, cancer marker blood tests that are often used in standard oncology, such as the prostate-specific-antigen (PSA, which is used to test for prostate cancer), ovarian CA-125 (for ovarian cancer), and the 15–3 and 19–9 (for breast cancer), do not always necessarily indicate whether you have cancer.

In my clinical experience, I have seen patients with normal cancer markers according to standardized cancer marker tests, but who do not yet have cancer. I also have seen patients whose cancer markers are falsely elevated due to the presence of an ovarian cyst or some other problem in the body.

In fact, the man who invented the PSA test, Richard J. Ablin, a research professor of immunobiology and pathology at the University of Arizona College of Medicine, has pointed out the shortcomings of the PSA in detecting prostate cancer. In an article published in the *New York Times* in 2010, Ablin writes about the PSA test: "As I've been trying to make clear for many years now, PSA testing can't detect prostate cancer and, more importantly, it can't distinguish between the two types of prostate cancer—the one that will kill you and the one that won't." He goes on to say, "In approving the procedure, the Food and Drug Administration relied heavily on a study that showed testing could detect 3.8 percent of prostate cancers, which was a better rate than the standard method, a digital rectal exam."[5]

This is why we recommend that you and your doctor use the other tests described earlier in this chapter, because they can be of great value for detecting cancer from the earliest stages, before the cancer has become dangerous and a potential disaster to your body. The Color Doppler Ultrasound and MRIs are important prostate cancer detection techniques.[6]

Early Symptoms That May Indicate Cancer

Certain symptoms can sometimes serve as small physical clues that cancer may be present in the body. These tend to show up before the disease manifests itself more aggressively. Most doctors miss these signs. If you have many or all of the following symptoms, and have not already been diagnosed with another medical condition, you may want to ask your doctor to test you for cancer.

The symptoms include:

- Failing eyesight (along with other signs, and not just as a symptom of aging)
- An attack of serious indigestion (gastrointestinal issues with symptoms consistent with bloating, constipation, acid reflux, etc.), which can be the first sign of cancer, and is caused by a blood clot in the pancreas. The clot reduces pancreatic function by 10 to 75 percent and leads to a short supply of pancreatic enzymes. This in turn may allow for tumors to grow because pancreatic enzymes control cancer cell growth in the body.
- Chronic fatigue. This is a characteristic shared by most cancer patients.
- Brain fog, or fuzzy thinking; a loss of clarity of thought
- Changes in the hair, especially hair that becomes brittle, coarse, balding, and graying
- Hernia, which is a symptom of many malignancies
- A peculiar body odor that doesn't wash away. Others may think of it as a "sickroom smell," or just "death."
- Muscle pains, particularly in the back and shoulders
- Palpable lumps, swelling, unusual bleeding, or any other symptom that is new and that doesn't resolve quickly on its own

The table Summary of Cancer Screening Tests (page 31) lists all the tests described in this chapter. By studying this table, you and your doctor can compare and contrast the different types of cancer screening tools available, to determine the ones that are best for you. If your doctor suspects that you have cancer, or you want to measure your progress on a cancer treatment regimen, it's a good idea to do multiple types of testing.

SUMMARY OF CANCER SCREENING TESTS

Cancer Prevention and Screening Tests	What the Test Measures	Purpose	How to Get It
The Cancer Profile	Nonspecific tumor markers, such as HCG, PHI, CEA, and DHEA sulfate	Detects cancer in the earliest stages: 10–12 years before tumor becomes detectable on other tests. A good cancer prevention test.	Order at www.American MetabolicLaboratories .net). No prescription needed.
ONCOblot	Looks for a protein called ENOX2 that exists only on the surface of cancer cells	Detects cancer 7–8 years before a tumor is detectable on other tests. A good cancer prevention test or can be used to determine whether cancer is present.	Order at www.ONCOblotlabs .com. A doctor's prescription is needed.
Research Genetic Cancer Center	Circulating tumor cells (CTCs) and circulating stem cells (CSCs)	Does a genetic analysis of cancer markers and will test cancer's sensitivity to a variety of natural and chemo agents. Also gives treatment recommendations based on genetics of cancer.	Order at www.RGCCusa. com. A doctor's prescription is needed. To find a doctor in the US that does RGCC testing, see http://www.rgccusa .com/doctor-locator/.
Thermography	Patterns of inflammation in the body; of vein patterns in the breast	For the prevention and detection of breast cancer. Also a marker of progress on treatment regimens.	Your doctor can order this test. Or to find a doctor that does this type of testing, see International Academy of Clinical Thermology: http:// www.iact-org .org/links.html.
I Sensitivity C-Reactive Protein	Nonspecific marker of inflammation	To help determine whether inflammation is present or environment in body is favorable to cancer development or progression.	Order via your doctor or online at such labs as www .labtestsonline.org. No prescription needed.
Hemoglobin A1C	Measures average blood sugar levels over 3 months	To determine whether environment in body is favorable to development of cancer or progression of cancer.	Order via your doctor or online at such labs as www .labtestsonline.org. No prescription needed.
Bioenergetic Testing	Looks for energy imbalances in the body	To discover the specific supportive treatments, nutrition and supplements that the body needs.	Ask for a practitioner recommendation at ZYTO. com or via integrative practitioner websites, such as www.ACAM.com or www.ACIM.com. (Also see Resources.)

continues

SUMMARY OF CANCER SCREENING TESTS   continued

Cancer Prevention and Screening Tests	What the Test Measures	Purpose	How to Get It
BioMeridian Testing	Uses acupuncture points to determine how energy is flowing throughout the body's meridian pathways or energy channels	Indicates inflammation, or to what extent there is deficiency and degeneration of organs. Can reveal how far along a person is in 12-year cancer development process.	Ask for a practitioner recommendation at Alternatives for Healing medical directory: http://www.alternatives forhealing.com/. (Also see Resources.)
PET Scan	Uses radiation to produce 3-D images of functional processes in the body	To see where tumors are in the body and the extent of illness (metastases).	Order via your doctor's prescription and do at your local hospital/clinic.

JACK'S Story

Jack's story suggests a perfect example of how using multiple diagnostic tests for cancer can make a world of difference. Jack had been seeking care at an integrative clinic for years—even before he began experiencing suspicious pain in his abdomen.

First, Jack did a PET scan, which could detect any potential cancer unless it was small. So instead, he had blood work and an abdominal ultrasound done to look at his pancreas, but his results all came out perfect. After that, he used a Cancer Profile test, and it showed elevated PHI enzymes, which indicated he had anaerobic metabolism—a sign that cancer could be present. He completed a circulating tumor cell test (CTC) from RGCC, and the results were 3.97, which isn't too high but still indicated possible cancer.

Finally, he did an ONCOblot test, which was the ultimate test that suggested he had cancer specifically in his pancreas. So, while two of the tests provided clues that he might have cancer, the ONCOblot confirmed the presence of the cancer. As a final step, he completed a BioMeridian test to definitively confirm the ONCOblot findings.

He immediately began taking pancreatic enzymes, which are special enzymes that contain such things as pancreatin, amylase, and lipase. Jack could tell right away that they were working because he felt better immediately. He is now taking the enzymes as part of a comprehensive, personalized wellness protocol, and he is recovering well.

CHAPTER 3

Groundbreaking Cancer Treatments

IN THIS CHAPTER, YOU WILL LEARN . . .

- The first steps you should take after you receive a cancer diagnosis
- Common cancer treatments used by integrative oncologists
- How to formulate a plan that fits your needs

"You have cancer" is among the most frightening phrases any of us could ever possibly hear, but cancer doesn't have to be a death sentence. You can often manage cancer like a chronic illness, or win your cancer battle and live for many years, working with an experienced and skilled integrative doctor alongside your current doctor. Many doctors now do long-distance telephone or Skype consults as well as in-person visits, so you can schedule a consult with a competent physician, no matter where you are, and receive guidance about the types of tests and treatments that would most benefit you. For more information about how to find a doctor and set yourself up for success, see Chapter 10.

In this chapter, you will learn about treatments that I believe can help patients battling cancer. Most skilled integrative cancer doctors will use a combination of at least some of these treatments, along with perhaps others, so we highly recommend working with a physician who is at least familiar with them, and ideally, knowledgeable and experienced in their use.

Not all of the following treatments will be useful or effective for treating the particular type of cancer that you have, but many can be. Your RGCC and other test results can help you and your doctor determine which of these would be best for you.

Not every late-stage cancer patient who does these treatments will be able to attain remission; however, I have seen many stage 3 and 4 cancer patients who have lived for years beyond their original prognoses, where they effectively combined these treatments into a comprehensive, individualized protocol. It's possible to unravel the whole twelve-year process that causes cancer in the first place. You may find that the treatments will enable you to do so as well if your doctors know how to use, combine, and integrate them into an effective treatment regimen.

For example, I have one patient, a sixty-six-year-old attorney who works full time and has stage 4 prostate cancer. The cancer is also in his ribs, but relatively speaking, he's doing great. You wouldn't think that he has a single thing wrong with him! However, some of our patients also do conventional treatments, and for those who do it seems like the more of those treatments that they do the worse they get. I'm not saying you shouldn't do conventional treatments, such as full-dose chemotherapy and radiation, because these treatments are sometimes appropriate and necessary, but if your doctor recommends them, you'll want to do therapies to support and heal your body at the same time, because chemotherapy harms the body and you and your doctor need to support your body to prevent it from being harmed.[1]

Another reason you'll want to collaborate with an integrative doctor is they can help you determine how effective conventional therapies alone may be. Unfortunately, some traditional oncologists tend to offer treatment advice based solely on a standard rulebook and suggest the same, inflexible treatment regimen for every patient who has a certain type of cancer—regardless of his or her unique characteristics. The truth is, ultimately, no doctor should ever be allowed to pronounce an "expiration date" on a patient because not only are we all individuals, but also, miracles do happen. Not to mention, there are many cases of spontaneous remission. No doctor—no one—knows when it's a person's time to die, but if doctors plant negative words into their patients, then negative things will be more likely to happen to them.

You'll want to work with a team of medical professionals who will give you hope, direct positive energy toward you, and encourage you in your fight against cancer. At the same time, I would recommend finding a doctor who uses at least some of the cutting-edge treatments that are described in this chapter. Again, see Chapter 10 for more information about how to find such a doctor and put together a supportive, successful team.

Throughout this chapter, I also list organizations that are specifically dedicated to providing information about some of the treatments that I describe here, and which maintain databases where you can also search for doctors who do that particular treatment.

What Happens When You First Visit an Integrative Cancer Clinic

Next, I'll describe the process our patients go through when they first come to our clinic. We encourage you to use this as a model to refer to when you are researching doctors or visiting clinics, to get a better idea about the kind of intake procedure and evaluation process that you should expect to find at a successful integrative cancer clinic.

The first thing we ask each patient to do is complete a medical questionnaire. Then, we have them set up a personal consultation with an integrative cancer specialist. That might be me, or another doctor on our team. As part of the consultation, we do a comprehensive clinical evaluation, which includes routine and extensive blood testing, along with the appropriate cancer detection tests, such as a PET scan, ONCOblot, Cancer Profile, CTCs, circulating tumor cells, or any of the others described in Chapter 2.

When evaluating our patients, we don't just look at the type or stage of their cancer. We consider many other factors, such as their age, other coexisting medical conditions, levels of environmental toxicity, infections (including viral, bacterial, parasitic, and fungal infections); and other treatments that they are doing, as well as the treatment plans that their other doctors have recommended.

We then have each patient meet with our nutritionist, Liliana Partida, who creates a specific, customized nutritional plan for them, consisting of foods that can act as medicines and help create an anticancer environment in the body. We also educate them on any necessary lifestyle changes and help them discover uplifting activities that will facilitate their treatment. In *The Cancer Revolution*, you will find guidelines for a healthy anticancer diet that are based on Liliana's recommendations.

As part of the process, we encourage our patients to see cancer as a wake-up call and tell them they must be willing to discard old diets, habits, and thoughts, and believe in the treatment path they have chosen for their treatments to be successful. They must be willing to give up their old way of living: whatever they were doing or not doing that was causing them to get sick in the first place.

We invite them to ask us questions and we make it clear that we want them to be fully involved in all of their treatment decisions. We try to help them see cancer as a challenge rather than a threat, and encourage them to focus on what they can do to make a difference in their wellness process. It is essential that you find a doctor and support system that will do the same for you, and encourage your feedback and participation in your recovery.

Finally, we don't just talk to our patients about the treatments that we do at our clinic, but we also discuss the types of traditional treatments that are available to them. We tell them about the benefits, as well as the side effects, that they can expect if they choose to do those treatments. We recommend that they see an oncologist in addition to us, so that they are well informed about all of the options that are available to them. A good integrative doctor won't be biased against conventional medicine, but will know how to pre-scribe it appropriately and not over- or underutilize it.

As discussed, conventional medicine has risks that your doctor needs to be able to discuss with you. Surgery, for example, has the potential to spread cancer cells into other areas of the body,[2] is no guarantee of a cure, and can be a traumatic event for the body and nervous system. Nonetheless, surgery may be the best option. If patients decide to undergo surgery, we recommend preparing the body two and a half weeks prior to the operation, and they have to be taken care of afterward.

It is also sometimes appropriate for patients to do full-dose chemotherapy and radiation, but these treatments also carry risks. For instance, they kill all types of cells: healthy cells *as well as* cancer cells. They compromise the immune system, and in some cases can severely sicken the patient.[3] Cancer cells can also develop resistance to chemotherapy, and in response to treat-ment, may mutate and create new types of cancer cells with a different, more treatment-resistant genetic makeup. Further, as science has fallen short on this front overall, conventional treatments can't eliminate circulating tumor cells (CTCs) and cancer stem cells (CSCs), which are responsible for 95 per-cent of all metastases.[4]

This is partially why the five-year survival rates for patients whose cancer has metastasized and who are treated exclusively with these methods is as low as it is: only 2 to 4 percent for lung, liver, prostate, stomach, pancreas, and esophageal cancers, and 11 to 30 percent for cancers of the kidney, colon, breast, ovary, and rectum, as well as melanomas.[5] Those shockingly low figures suggest the standard of care in cancer treatment today is woefully inadequate.

However, as I mentioned, chemotherapy and radiation do have their place in cancer treatment, and integrative doctors do a form of low-dose chemotherapy called IPT that may be more effective than full-dose chemotherapy for some patients. And yet at other times, it is recommended that some of our patients see an oncologist to receive full-dose chemotherapy because a few types of cancer (testicular and lymphoma) respond well to it.

Regardless of the treatment path you choose, your doctor should always customize your regimen to your individual needs because no two patients are the same. Your doctor should also change and rotate your regimen over time because cancer will often develop resistance to the same treatments and it's important to continually outsmart it.

Something else that many integrative doctors emphasize is once patients have cancer and have effectively treated it, they must still do follow-up testing for the rest of their life, and continue to monitor and manage it like a chronic illness. Many of our patients have already received conventional treatments, and were told by their doctors that they were cancer free, only to hear the words "You have stage 4 cancer" (again!)—two, three, or five years later. So, once you know that you are susceptible to cancer, you have to continue to do things to stay well, such as maintain a healthy diet and lifestyle, and do follow-up testing periodically. We have found, for instance, that some of our patients need follow-up testing every six months, while others need to be continually monitored, with follow-up testing as often as every three months.

Groundbreaking Cancer Treatments

Insulin Potentiation Targeted Low-Dose Chemotherapy

Insulin potentiation targeted low-dose chemotherapy (IPT, a.k.a. IPTLD) is a form of low-dose chemotherapy that many integrative doctors give their patients to shrink a tumor mass. IPT is great because usually patients experience few to no side effects from it.[6] So, unlike patients who do full-dose chemotherapy, those who do IPT don't experience hair loss, vomiting, and other side effects. Often, cancer patients can maintain a high quality of life during IPT treatment.

This simple medical procedure involves intravenously administering the hormone insulin to the body, followed by glucose and various anticancer agents. For this procedure, we use one tenth of the traditional chemotherapy dose, using specific anticancer agents that test best for each patient, according to RGCC testing.

Here's the logic behind IPT: Cancer cells have ten times more insulin receptors on their surface than does a regular cell. Insulin is a hormone that your body uses to shuttle glucose into the cells. So, when you give your body insulin, along with glucose, the insulin acts as a "Trojan horse" or an escort, to more effectively bring not only glucose but also the anticancer agents into the cancer cells. Because some studies suggest sugar may fuel the growth of cancer,[7] they readily open up the insulin receptors and "eat" the glucose, along with the chemotherapy drugs and/or natural anticancer agents.

Insulin also helps the body fight cancer because it prompts cancer cells to divide, which is when they are most vulnerable to being destroyed by drugs and other anticancer agents. Experts in the field of integrative oncology believe insulin does this during what is called the "therapeutic moment"— when your blood sugar has been lowered enough for the chemotherapy to be administered most effectively. Because normal cells don't have as many insulin receptors as cancer cells, they don't absorb very much of the glucose or the chemotherapy agents, which means that patients aren't likely to suffer severe side effects from it.

IPT was developed in 1930 and has been used by integrative cancer doctors since 1946, so it is not a new therapy, and studies have suggested its effectiveness. For instance, one study on breast cancer patients at George Washington University found that using insulin, along with the breast chemotherapy drug methotrexate, increased the killing effect of the methotrexate by a factor of ten thousand.[8]

IPT has been reported among some integrative doctors to work especially well for breast, prostate, lung, colon, bladder, uterine, and stomach cancers, as well as for lymphomas, sarcomas, and melanomas. There are even reports that suggest IPT has helped send some cancers, such as pancreatic, ovarian, and renal cell cancers, into remission. Other cancers that studies suggest respond well to IPT include blood, bone, cervical, and esophageal cancers. Unlike traditional full-dose chemotherapy, IPT is thought to produce few to no side effects. Some patients become slightly anemic or tired from it, but in general, most usually tolerate it well.

For more information about IPT and to find doctors that do IPT, see the Resources section at the end of this book.

Insulin-Potentiated High-Dose IV Vitamin C

Researchers have discovered that when vitamin C is given to the body intravenously in large doses, it has oxidative, rather than antioxidant effects, and can be selectively toxic to cancer cells. Within tumors, vitamin C generates large amounts of hydrogen peroxide, which is lethal to cancer cells. At the same time, intravenous vitamin C doesn't damage healthy tissue because healthy cells produce high amounts of catalase, which is an enzyme that neutralizes hydrogen peroxide, so that the hydrogen peroxide can't damage the cells. However, most cancers don't produce much catalase, which means that they can't defend themselves against the toxic hydrogen peroxide that vitamin C produces. Also, like its use in IPT, insulin can be used to more effectively drive vitamin C into cancer cells.

The vitamin C–hydrogen peroxide–catalase connection was first discovered by Dr. Mark Levine, an internationally acclaimed researcher at the National Institutes of Health, who led a team of researchers to analyze the cancer-killing effects of high-dose vitamin C treatment. But it was actually the Nobel Prize–winning scientist Dr. Linus Pauling, along with British cancer surgeon Ewan Cameron, who were the first to discover and use vitamin C treatment for terminal cancer patients, in the 1970s.

In two published clinical trials, Drs. Pauling and Cameron reported that vitamin C significantly prolonged and improved their patients' quality of lives.[9] For these trials, Pauling and Cameron used mega-doses of 10 grams (10,000 mg) of IV vitamin C, followed by an additional 10 grams of oral vitamin C. In later years, C. G. Moertel, MD, conducted controlled clinical studies at the Mayo Clinic and reported in the *New England Journal of Medicine* that he was unable to replicate the results of Drs. Pauling and Cameron.[10]

Because of Dr. Moertel's studies, for years many health professionals disregarded high-dose vitamin C as a viable treatment option for their patients. Yet recently, researchers from the National Institutes of Health have begun investigating vitamin C again because new research may indicate that Drs. Pauling and Cameron were right.

Dr. Levine, who discovered the vitamin C–hydrogen peroxide–catalase connection, believed that Dr. Moertel's trials failed because he only gave his subjects vitamin C orally, while research suggests dozens of grams of vitamin C must be given intravenously for it to work. Oral vitamin C is completely ineffective against cancer. This is because the effect that vitamin C has upon the body depends upon the dose that is taken.[11] At low doses, it has anti-oxidative effects upon the body; at high doses, it has oxidant, or cancer-killing effects. In fact, there are many substances that render very different effects upon the body, depending on the dosage. The difference between a venom and cure is often in the amount. It's hard to believe, but even drinking too much water can kill you. We and other integrative doctors have treated hundreds of patients with high-dose vitamin C, and found it to be both safe and effective.

Yet this therapy hasn't worked for everyone, and a few variables can undermine its effectiveness. The fact that some tumors produce larger amounts of catalase than others, which neutralizes the cancer-killing effects of hydrogen peroxide, is one variable. Also, sometimes there is an insufficient amount of oxygen in the space around the cells, which is needed for vitamin C to produce hydrogen peroxide.

For now, scientists have not found a way to stop tumors from producing catalase. However, we have found that adding vitamin K_3 to our patients' vitamin C IVs markedly increases the creation of hydrogen peroxide in some tumors, enabling a more substantial "kill" in those cancers that have high catalase activity. Vitamin K_3 is a synthetic form of vitamins K_1 and K_2. In integrative medicine, it is often used before and after administering low-dose chemotherapy because it can also prevent metastases, or the spreading of cancer to other tissues and organs. Patients usually experience no side effects from this treatment.

Many integrative doctors do IV vitamin C treatments. You can find one in your area by doing a practitioner search at one of the medical association websites listed in Chapter 10 and in the Resources section at the end of this book. The popular cancer information site CancerTutor.com also maintains a list of a few doctors that do IV vitamin C.

Supportive Oligonucleotide Technique

Supportive oligonucleotide technique (SOT) uses oligonucleotides, the short chains of a cancer's DNA or RNA molecules, to bind and inactivate what is called "messenger RNA" (mRNA), which is a gene product produced by cancer cells. This has the effect of turning cancer genes "off," which then disables the cancer. In other words, SOT uses messenger RNA to negatively influence the genetic expression of the cancer. We have been using SOT at our clinic since about August 2013, but it has been used in Europe for many years. Currently there are few clinics in the United States that offer this type of treatment, but hopefully that will change in the years to come.

SOT is an intravenous treatment that is formulated by Research Genetic Cancer Center (RGCC) lab. RGCC analyzes the mRNA (a genetic component) of your circulating tumor cells (CTCs) and cancer stem cells (CSCs), and then creates the SOT treatment based on your specific cancer gene patterns, as well as occasionally from biopsies of the tumor(s). SOT causes CTCs, CSCs, and tumor cancer cells to self-destruct in a process called apoptosis. The end goal of this technique is to reduce the number of CTCs and CSCs in the body and to establish tumor stability so the tumor doesn't continue to grow and reproduce out of control.

This treatment works around the clock, 24/7, and can be combined with other therapies. It works in the body for sixteen to eighteen weeks, after which time you can receive another intravenous infusion. The general standard is patients can receive up to three infusions per year. There are no known side effects from SOT.[12] To find a practitioner in your state or country that does SOT, I would recommend contacting RGCC for a referral or doing a practitioner search at one of the medical organization websites listed in the Resources.

Autohemotherapy

Autohemotherapy involves briefly removing 100 to 200 ml of blood from the body and exposing it to ultraviolet light and ozone. For this procedure, blood is withdrawn from the patient's arm using an IV needle and tubing. (The exact amount taken depends upon the patient's body weight.) The blood is then run through a device that exposes it to controlled ultraviolet rays and ozone. Once it has been exposed to the light and ozone, it is shuttled back into the bloodstream.

Some integrative doctors use an advanced type of autohemotherapy called the UVL(RX) Treatment System, which delivers light therapy intravenously without having to remove the blood from the patient's body. UVL(RX) is an improvement over traditional autohemotherapy because it allows doctors to treat nearly 100 percent of their patients' blood, unlike standard auto-hemotherapy that only treats a small percentage. It also is safer because the blood doesn't need to be removed from the body.

Both standard autohemotherapy and improved forms of autohemotherapy, such as the UVL(RX) Treatment System, can help you battle cancer indirectly, by removing the factors that are causing your immune system to be suppressed. Among its many benefits, autohemotherapy can:

- Inactivate cancer-causing toxins
- Destroy and inhibit bacterial, fungal, and viral growth in the bloodstream
- Bring oxygen to the organs. Remember, cancer cells don't like oxygen!
- Activate the production of steroid hormones, which assist the immune system in fighting cancer
- Stimulate the immune system and activate the white blood cells, so that the body can more effectively identify and kill the cancer
- Stimulate fibrinolysis, which is the process that the body uses to break up blot clots
- Decrease the viscosity, or thickness of the blood, and increase tissue oxygenation and microcirculation. This enables treatments to reach the cancer cells more easily and be more effective.
- Reduce inflammation so that the immune system can function better
- Improve the body's tolerance to radiation and chemotherapy

Generally, people experience no side effects from this therapy. To find a doctor who does autohemotherapy and/or uses the UVL(RX) Treatment System, see the Resources.

Hyperbaric Oxygen Therapy

Hyperbaric oxygen therapy (HBOT) is a well-established treatment for cancer and other diseases, whereby the patient lies down and breathes pure oxygen through a mask inside of a sealed chamber, while the pressure inside of the chamber is slowly raised to two to three times that of the normal atmosphere. At this pressure, oxygen, which is normally delivered to the tissues through the body's hemoglobin in the red blood cells, is dissolved in all of the body fluids, including the plasma (which is the pale yellow liquid component of blood that normally holds the blood cells in suspension); and the cerebrospinal fluid in the brain, spinal cord, and lymph.

This oxygen is then transported to all of the tissues. With HBOT, the cells receive fifteen times more oxygen than they would under normal conditions, and the lungs can gather up to three times more oxygen than they otherwise would by breathing in a normal environment. HBOT is medicine's most efficient method of transporting oxygen throughout the body.

HBOT can help your body fight cancer in a number of ways. Cancer cells hate oxygen and survive in an anaerobic environment, so when they are exposed to high levels of oxygen, they are more susceptible to death. HBOT can also substantially repair healthy cells, and can stimulate your body to release growth factors and stem cells that promote healing. Additionally, it has been shown to significantly reduce inflammation. Many doctors use it on patients who have received radiation therapy, to reduce inflammation in the bones and adjacent tissues because radiation damages these parts of the body.

A patient's hyperbaric oxygen sessions can be combined with nutraceutical supplements (products that are derived from food sources) and a medication called Trental (pentoxifylline), which thins the blood and enhances blood flow and oxygenation to the tissues. This procedure is called oxidative preconditioning therapy.

The effects of a ninety-minute HBOT session last four to five hours. We often follow up our patients' HBOT sessions with a treatment called pulsed electromagnetic field (PEMF) therapy, which further helps carry oxygen into the cancer cells. (For more information on PEMF, see page 46.) HBOT is used by some integrative doctors in the United States, as well as in Mexico and Europe. To find an HBOT clinic in your area, ask for a referral at the International Hyperbarics Association (internationalhyperbaricsassociation .org). Alternatively, you can find doctors who do HBOT by researching online at the medical association websites, especially ACAM.org. See the Resources for more information.

Ozone Therapy

Ozone therapy is similar to oxygen therapy but has somewhat different effects upon the body. Yet like oxygen, ozone is a well-established cancer treatment that helps the body heal in a variety of ways: it causes cancer cells to self-destruct; increases oxygen delivery to the cells, tissues, and organs; detoxifies the blood; increases blood circulation throughout the body; and boosts the immune system.

Ozone therapy can be administered in different ways, including vaginally and rectally. It also can be applied intravenously, which is the method I prefer based on my personal experience. For this procedure, a certain amount of blood is removed from the patient's body and then saturated with ozone. When ozone contacts the bloodstream it breaks down into oxygen. The doctor then puts that oxygen-rich blood back into the patient's body. Increasingly, integrative cancer clinics are doing ozone therapy as part of their patients' treatment regimens. People generally experience no side effects from ozone.

Intravenous Curcumin Therapy

Curcumin is an anti-inflammatory component of the popular South Asian spice turmeric, which is a member of the ginger family. It is also a powerful anticancer agent that counteracts some of the initial processes in the body that lead to cancer, as well as the mechanisms that allow tumors to grow and cancer to spread. Among its anticancer properties, curcumin interferes with the development of cancer stem cells, which are "baby" cancer cells that are not affected by traditional chemotherapy. It also enhances the effectiveness of certain types of chemotherapy when it is used prior to the therapy, and disrupts the production of NF-kappaB, an inflammatory chemical that is responsible for initiating the estimated twelve-year-long process that created the cancer in the first place.

Clinical trials involving curcumin have suggested it may be as effective as pharmaceutical drugs for treating all kinds of cancers.[13] In my experience, I have seen a patient who had suffered for five years from a rectal tumor that had extended into her colon—and caused her a lot of pain and uncomfortable bowel movements—until after just six treatments of IV curcumin, her pain dramatically diminished and her bowel movements normalized.

Taking curcumin intravenously is more beneficial than taking it by mouth, since it bypasses the stomach, which means that 100 percent of it gets absorbed by the body. It also works better and more quickly when given intravenously, and your physician can give you higher doses than you would otherwise be able to tolerate. Studies suggest curcumin isn't just beneficial for cancer but also for any inflammatory condition. You can ask your doctor to order curcumin from a compounding pharmacy, which he or she can then give to you via IV. People generally experience no side effects as a result of doing IV curcumin therapy.

Peptide Bioregulator Therapy

Peptide bioregulator therapy is designed to regenerate damaged organs, tissues, and systems in the body that have become dysfunctional or injured due to stress, toxins, and cancer. It involves taking, either orally or via injection, peptides from embryonic or young calves, sheep, pigs, and other animals, to stimulate the body to help revitalize and create new, healthy tissue. It does this by regulating genes that direct the creation of new cells. Different peptides are used, depending upon the organ, system, or tissue that needs to be regenerated. So, for instance, liver peptides from a young calf would be used to regenerate the liver, while heart peptide would be used to regenerate the heart.

Peptide bioregulator therapy is similar to live cell therapy, which was first discovered by the Swiss physician Paul Niehans in 1931, when he injected a solution containing ground-up parathyroid cells from a calf into a patient who had damaged parathyroid glands. The patient recovered, and according to anecdotal reports, Dr. Niehans then treated more than thirty thousand patients with live cells. He claimed that cancer patients who received live cell therapy were five times less likely to die than were those who didn't receive it.[14]

Peptide therapy is not yet widely available in the United States, but it is recognized and utilized as an adjunct cancer treatment in other integrative cancer clinics abroad. A company in Estonia offers bioregulator supplements without a prescription. These peptides are just as effective as live cell therapy injections, and have been developed over the last forty years by Professor Vladimir Khavinson, a world-renowned gerontologist and president of the European Association of Gerontology and Geriatrics. The former USSR government spent over $300 million to research and develop treatments that would promote longevity in their military. Professor Khavinson and his colleagues were involved in the research, and ended up developing a complicated method for extracting peptides from different animal tissues and synthesizing them into a form that would stimulate the body's own creation of new tissue.

Another benefit of peptides is they don't just regenerate the organs and tissues damaged by cancer; they also powerfully stimulate the immune system to help the body prevent and fight it. According to an interview with Professor Khavinson, in fifteen studies that were conducted on approximately three thousand animals, a thymus extract product called Vladonix was shown to decrease cancer risk by three- to fivefold. Studies have also shown the extract to extend the life span of mice by 30 to 40 percent.[15] Vladonix was developed in the 1970s, and so has a long history of use in Russia, particularly among former military members.

During my clinical practice, I have observed that peptides are safe and generally side effect free. Currently, the company that sells the products developed by Professor Khavinson, Senpai OÜ, has a website that contains published studies that demonstrate the potential long-term effects of the peptides for a variety of health conditions, including cancer.

Pulsed Electromagnetic Field Therapy

Pulsed electromagnetic field (PEMF) therapy uses a pulsed electromagnet to change cellular processes in the body and is thought to be a vital component of all our cancer treatment protocols. In integrative medicine, PEMF therapy is administrated to patients after they do IV vitamin C therapy and/or hyperbaric oxygen therapy because it enhances the effects of these therapies.

PEMF can provide a major energy boost to healthy cells, helping them uptake nutrients and get rid of waste. When the body can't eliminate waste from the cells, it's similar to having the garbage men on strike, so it's important to do things to eliminate it. PEMF helps the body detoxify while promoting proper cellular metabolism. PEMF can help restore cells to a normal, healthy, and balanced electrical state amid exposure to chemicals or otherwise undesirable toxins.

In people with cancer, PEMF also concentrates nutrients into the tumor area and encourages their destruction. Research has shown cancer cells function at a significantly lower electrical voltage than regular healthy cells, and so are weakened by electromagnetic stimulation. In 2011, the FDA approved PEMF therapy for the treatment of brain cancer. And a study published in 2006 suggested PEMF therapy helped shrink melanomas by 90 percent within two weeks of treatment.[16]

PEMF therapy is safe, painless, and noninvasive. It generally produces no side effects. Among its many other potential benefits, it can reduce pain, diminish inflammation, accelerate wound and injury healing, help the body grow new bone and neurons, improve gene and protein expression, restore the body's energetic balance, and reestablish proper cellular function and metabolism.

Many integrative doctors now use PEMF therapy as part of their cancer treatment. You may be able to find a doctor who does PEMF therapy by doing a search on one of the medical association websites listed in the Resources. Alternatively, ask for a practitioner referral from one of the companies or websites that sell PEMF devices or provide information on PEMF therapy. For more information and to contact these organizations, see the Resources. The website PEMF.com also contains studies that demonstrate the estimated effectiveness of PEMF therapy for a variety of conditions.

SUMMARY OF CANCER TREATMENTS

Cancer Treatments	How They Work	Where to Find Practitioners That Do Them*
Insulin Potentiation Targeted Low-Dose Chemotherapy (IPT)	• Uses insulin to drive chemotherapy and other anticancer agents more effectively into the cells, at one tenth of the normal chemotherapy dose	• Academy for Comprehensive Integrative Medicine: www.acim connect.com • American College for Advancement in Medicine: www.acam.org • International Organization of Integrative Cancer Physicians: www.ioicp.com • Best Answer for Cancer: www.bestanswerforcancer.org Also: www.IPTQ.com www.IPTforCancer.com
Insulin Potentiation High-Dose IV Vitamin C	• Creates hydrogen peroxide inside cancer cells, which is lethal to them • Uses insulin to more effectively drive vitamin C into the cells	See medical organizations listed above. Also: Cancer Tutor: http://www.cancertutor.com /vitaminc_ivc/
Supportive Oligonucleotide Technique (SOT)	• Uses short chains of DNA or RNA molecules to bind and inactivate mRNA, which turns cancer genes "off" • Causes circulating tumor cells (CTCs) and circulating stem cells (CSCs) to self-destruct	See medical organizations listed above. Also: www.rgcc-genlab.com
Autohemotherapy	• Encourages cancer cell self-destruction • Inactivates cancer-causing toxins • Inhibits pathogenic growth • Stimulates immune function • Increases oxygenation in tissues • Lowers inflammation • Increases tolerance to radiation and chemotherapy	• See medical organizations listed above. • For information on the UVL(RX) Treatment System, consult UVL(RX) Therapeutics: www.uvlrx.com.

continues

SUMMARY OF CANCER TREATMENTS continued

Cancer Treatments	How They Work	Where to Find Practitioners That Do Them*
Hyperbaric Oxygen Therapy (HBOT)	• Saturates tissues with oxygen, which is toxic to cancer cells, and helps healthy cells function better	See medical organizations listed on page 47. Also: International Hyperbarics Association, Inc.: http://www.ihausa.org/
IV Ozone	• Increases oxygen in the body, which is toxic to cancer cells but beneficial for healthy cells • Detoxifies the blood • Boosts immune function • Increases blood circulation	See medical organizations listed on page 47. Also: American Academy of Ozonotherapy: http://aaot.us/
IV Curcumin	• Disables tumor survival mechanisms and processes in the body that lead to cancer • Interferes with cancer stem cell development • Enhances effectiveness of chemotherapy • Disrupts NF-kappaB, an inflammatory chemical responsible for initiation of cancer development	See medical organizations listed on page 47.
Peptide Bioregulator Therapy	• Stimulates the body to produce new cells and regenerates sick, damaged, or weak organs	Can be purchased online at www.peptidesstore.com.
Pulsed Electromagnetic Field Therapy (PEMF)	• Detoxifies the body • Restores cells to a normal, balanced electrical state • Reduces pain and inflammation • Uses magnetic pulses to change the permeability of the cell wall. Allows for greater absorption of nutrients and elimination of waste. • Induces a charge around all the cells in the area of use. As cancer cells operate at a much lower voltage than healthy cells, it weakens their metabolic processes. • Acts to "un-clump" red and white blood cells, allowing greater circulation and pain relief	See medical organizations listed on page 47. To locate a practitioner with the stronger professional model, please visit www.pulse4life.com For home usage we recommend the MAS device. http://maswellness.com.

* At these organizations' websites you can search for physicians that do most of the treatments listed in this table.

The table of cancer treatments on pages 47–48 summarizes the principal treatments that I have described in this chapter, along with a brief explanation of how they can benefit the body. By studying this table, you will get a good idea about some of the best integrative cancer treatments out there; how these treatments support the body; and how you can either find a doctor who does the treatments, or cooperate with your doctor to access them.

NANCY'S Story

Nancy is a forty-six-year-old cancer patient who was diagnosed with stage 4 colon cancer that had spread to her liver and lymph nodes. She chose the conventional route of treatment, but she also sought supportive therapies because she understood she needed to help keep her body strong and as healthy as possible while undergoing chemotherapy. Those supplemental recommendations helped her attain the best possible outcome with her conventional treatment regimen.

Nancy's surgeon had told her that the survival rate for stage 4 colon cancer was less than 20 percent, so she consulted with several oncologists, and they all agreed she should do six months of chemotherapy followed by surgery and another six months of chemotherapy. She ended up having liver and colon surgery, and she sought alternative care at the same time she received chemotherapy from her oncologist. She used an arsenal of ammunition to help fortify her body, and she began exercising for thirty minutes a day, taking vitamins, and doing coffee enemas, infrared saunas, live cell therapy, wheatgrass shots and green juicing, among other things.

Nancy's blood work went back to normal so fast that her oncologist declared it was a miracle and said that he had never seen anything like it. It's been four years since her diagnosis, and Nancy's tumor markers are now normal, and she's doing remarkably well.

PART TWO

THE SIX REVOLUTIONARY CANCER STRATEGIES

CHAPTER 4

Let Food Be Your Medicine

IN THIS CHAPTER, YOU WILL DISCOVER . . .

- Which foods are medicine and which promote cancer growth
- The powerful anticancer benefits of a ketogenic (low carb, high fat, moderate protein)
- Lists of key foods that will enable you to fight cancer and feel your best

Did you know that what you eat and drink could be the single most important determinant of whether you develop cancer or beat it? The right foods are medicine for your body and contain all of the vital nutrients that you need to improve and function properly. We all want energy, and you need energy to fight cancer, but to get it, you need to have the proper types and proportions of protein, carbohydrates, and fatty foods in your diet, and to choose the sources of these macronutrients wisely and thoughtfully; otherwise, the machinery of your body won't run well.

The nutrients your body needs are not found in cookies, crackers, or macaroni and cheese! These are what I call "dead" foods. If you want to feel alive and be flooded with energy, you must eat real foods that are life-giving. Some people will argue that meat isn't life-giving, but this isn't true. If you study how hunter-gatherers in ancient societies used to eat, you'll find, for example, that whenever they had a problem with a specific organ or felt weak, they ate animal organs and these meats (or a broth made from them) strengthened them.

Meat, and especially organ meat, contains the genetic material that a weakened body needs to repair itself. Other life-giving foods include such things as fresh, organic vegetables, nuts, and healthy oils. In this chapter you'll learn more about such foods, as well as which foods you need to avoid because they steal life from your body.

How a Low-Carb, Moderate-Protein, High-Fat Food Plan Can Help Fight Cancer

Integrative doctors customize patients' food plans to their specific needs. At the same time, there are certain dietary principles that are recommended, and I describe those here. You'll want to share these with your doctor, too.

One type of anticancer food plan that is highly recommended is low in carbohydrates, moderate in protein, and high in healthy fat. It is sometimes known as a ketogenic diet. This type of diet changes the way the body uses energy. Normally, your body primarily uses glucose to create energy. Glucose comes from carbohydrates, so if you don't consume high amounts of carbohydrates, your body will resort to breaking down fat in a process called ketosis. In ketosis, your body creates what are called ketone bodies, which are compounds that your liver produces when it breaks down fat and uses it, instead of glucose, as an energy source. Because cancer cells use glucose for energy but can't use ketone bodies, a ketogenic diet is thought to help starve them.

For your body to use fat for energy and go into ketosis, you must consume very few carbohydrate-containing foods in your diet. This doesn't have to be a painful process. The ketogenic food plan provides an ample amount of calories from fat and protein, so you generally don't feel hungry on it. And normal, healthy cells can effectively utilize either glucose or ketones for energy, so many people feel great on this type of a food plan once they adapt to it. It is also great because it's anti-inflammatory and benefits your gut. This happens because the diet eliminates any allergenic or fungal-forming foods. Plus, it's high in good, healthy fats, which can improve your cell membranes. That piece is important because your cell membranes are the "gatekeepers" that allow nutrients into your cells, and at the same time they enable waste to be more effectively removed from them.

Foods that comprise a ketogenic diet include low-glycemic (or low sugar), nonstarchy green, leafy vegetables; organic, grass-fed, non-GMO animal protein products, such as eggs, seafood, poultry, beef, and other meats; and healthy fats, such as almonds, and olive and coconut oil. In general, most green, leafy vegetables, such as asparagus, spinach, kale, cauliflower, cabbage, lettuce, and collard greens, are permitted on the diet. Most higher-glycemic vegetables, such as potatoes, beets, and winter squash, are not.

A wealth of research suggests the ketogenic diet can aid in cancer prevention and assist the body in warding off the disease among people diagnosed with it. For instance, in 2012, researcher Dr. Thomas Seyfried, professor of neurogenetics and neurochemistry at Yale University and Boston College, wrote a book that describes the biochemistry of cancer and how it works, and concluded that the ketogenic diet is the best type of diet for unraveling cancer and defeating its survival mechanisms.[1] His book, entitled *Cancer as a Metabolic Disease: On the Origin, Management, and Prevention of Cancer*, expands upon the theories of Otto Warburg, MD, a great German scientist who won a Nobel Prize in Physiology or Medicine in 1931 for discovering that cancer cells get their food through glycolysis (by fermenting glucose without oxygen).[2]

According to Dr. Seyfried, when you follow a low-carb, or ketogenic, diet and restrict the amount of calories that you consume, your body goes into a metabolic state that is hostile to cancer cells.[3] The idea behind the ketogenic diet is because cancer needs glucose to thrive, and carbohydrates turn to glucose in your body, you can help starve cancer by simply limiting your consumption of carbohydrate-containing foods.

For your body to burn ketones rather than glucose for energy, you need to find out what your carbohydrate threshold is. This is the maximum amount of carbohydrates you can eat and still burn fat for energy. Knowing your personal threshold is important because your body will not revert to burning ketones for energy unless your carbohydrate consumption is below a certain level, and some people can consume higher amounts of carbohydrates on a ketogenic diet than others.

Perhaps you've heard of metabolic-typing diets, which are based on the premise that we are unique and convert food into energy differently, and therefore we need different combinations of healthy foods. For instance, based on the principles of metabolic typing, some people are what are called "fast cellular oxidizers," while others are "slow cellular oxidizers." This simply means that some people burn carbohydrates and convert food into energy faster than others do. Fast oxidizers—people who are fast burners—tolerate fewer carbohydrates on a low-carb food plan than do those who are slow oxidizers. This is because in fast oxidizers, carbohydrates hit the bloodstream faster and cause blood sugar spikes more readily than in people who are slow oxidizers.

According to one of my colleagues, who establishes nutritional food plans for patients, if you are a "fast oxidizer," you may only be able to tolerate as few as 10 grams of carbohydrates per day on a ketogenic diet, whereas slow oxidizers might be able to consume 30 to 40 grams daily on the diet. A green salad or twelve spears of asparagus might contain only 9 to 10 grams of carbohydrates, but for some people, this will be sufficient when they add in animal protein and ample amounts of fatty foods to their diet. In the Recipes section of the book, we share some low-carb ketogenic recipes you can make at home if you wish to try out this diet.

The ketogenic diet is best done under physician supervision, so if you decide to pursue this diet, it's a good idea to work with an integrative or holistic cancer doctor who understands it, or who is at least open to learning about it. Increasingly, integrative cancer doctors are recommending a low-carb food plan to their patients, so it shouldn't be too difficult to find one who can help you do it. It's also a good idea to consult with a doctor because, although this diet has significant anticancer benefits, it isn't for everyone, so you'll want to find out first whether it's the best type of diet for your particular body chemistry.

In the meantime, you can read more about the ketogenic diet by consulting one of the many books on ketogenic diets that are out there, such as Jimmy Moore's *Keto Clarity: Your Definitive Guide to the Benefits of a Low-Carb, High-Fat Diet,* as it is beyond the scope of this book to describe the intricacies of the diet in detail.

For patients who follow this type of low-carb food plan, once their health has stabilized, I have found they can increase their carbohydrate intake from 10 to 30 grams daily to 40 to 60 grams daily, an amount that is sufficiently low to keep the cancer from recurring, but high enough so that they can incorporate some additional higher-carbohydrate foods into their diet if they wish. These include berries or healthy dairy products, such as non-GMO goat's milk yogurt or goat cheese. Berries and yogurt can help the body detoxify, and yogurt is healing to the gastrointestinal tract.

The ketogenic food plan is similar to what our ancestors used to eat—a healthy caveman diet—and when it's balanced with enough green vegetables, it is beneficial for many people. Of course, I have observed that some patients fare better on other types of diets, such as a plant-based or vegetarian diet, which is comprised of plant protein, supplemental amino acids, and higher amounts of healthy vegetables. These diets are also relatively low in carbohydrates, but might contain more or different varieties of vegetables, and/or perhaps some low glycemic fruits and small amounts of healthy dairy products. The types of amino acids that we give our patients are highly bioavailable to the body, and are described later in this chapter.

In any case, you'll want to work with a good integrative doctor who understands nutrition to determine the diet that's best for you, or first try out some of the recipes at the end of this book to see how you feel. Most of our patients do well by following these recipes, or will only need to make small adjustments to them, to reap their benefits. The 14-day plan in Chapter 12 will also help you implement a ketogenic-based eating plan.

One way to confirm that you are eating the right foods or combinations of foods is to test your body's pH. Later in this chapter, I describe pH and a simple, do-it-yourself home test for measuring yours.

Regardless of whether you choose to pursue a low-carb food plan, if there's one rule I'd recommend abiding by, it is to eliminate sugar and all foods that metabolically turn to sugar in your body. These include higher-glycemic fruits, bread, rice, white potatoes, pastries, pasta, popcorn, and crackers. Minimizing carbs is thought to be one of the most foundational principles of any healthy anticancer diet.

Eating well doesn't have to be a chore or complicated, though. You mostly just want to eat foods that are produced according to the rules of Mother Nature: fresh, natural, and unprocessed. When you discover how great real foods will make you feel, and all the life-giving benefits that you'll experience from them, I think you'll find that a low-carb, anticancer diet isn't drudgery or difficult to do.

Your pH and the Benefits of Keeping Your Body Alkaline

You've probably heard about pH before. This is a measure of how acidic or alkaline your body is. Every food you eat will either cause your body to become more acidic or more alkaline. All junk and most processed foods, for example, will make you acidic. It's important to discover how different foods affect your pH because your body's pH can have a lot to do with whether you will recover from cancer and the likelihood that you will be able to prevent it. You want your pH to be balanced, at a level of 7.4, which is neutral—neither too acidic nor too alkaline—because cancer thrives in an environment that is either too acidic or too alkaline (most cancers prefer an acidic environment, however).

For this reason, when putting together a food plan, you don't want to look just at what foods could aid in starving your cancer or make you feel good, but also what foods and combinations of foods will help balance your pH. Most of us are too acidic because we aren't eating the right foods or combinations of foods. We are also acidic because of stress and environmental toxins because acidity isn't just caused by eating the wrong foods, but also the toll our daily lives can take on our body.

When you become acidic, it creates a condition in your body called acidosis. When the body is in acidosis, it doesn't work properly. It's basically paralyzed and functioning at half of its total capacity. It's like having a sail at half-mast that won't get you to where you want to go, or putting a substance other than gasoline into your car. Our body thrives when all of our 100 trillion cells are effectively communicating with one another. They do this through chemical, electrical, and hormonal processes, but when they become too acidic, then this communication doesn't happen . . . and pretty soon, none of our organs or systems works well.

The body has a wonderful mechanism for eliminating the excess acids produced by acidosis. It does this by drawing upon alkalizing minerals, such as magnesium, sodium, and calcium, which are stored in the organs and bones. These minerals neutralize the harmful acids, but over time, this creates mineral deficiencies that can lead to such problems as osteoporosis, as minerals get progressively leeched from the bones. Also, the body may not be able to keep up with the demand for minerals, and can become overwhelmed and unable to eliminate the excess acid. In an effort to protect the vital organs, it will store the excess harmful acids in the tissues, joints, and bones, which then causes pain and all kinds of musculoskeletal and tissue problems.

When acidosis exists over long term, it creates many other problems, such as inflammation, reduced white blood cell production, damaged cells and cell membranes, and cells that make "mistakes" as they try to repair and regenerate themselves. This creates a prime environment for cancer and all kinds of degenerative diseases. There is also less oxygen available to the cells, and by now you know that cancer thrives in a low oxygen-environment. Microorganisms also reproduce in a low-oxygen environment, so acidosis makes it possible for fungi, yeast, parasites, bacteria, and viruses to flourish and weaken your immune system so that it can't effectively fight the cancer.

By measuring your pH, you can find out whether you are on track with your diet. It is easy to do this. First, purchase some saliva pH strips, which you can get from your local pharmacy or an online retailer. The strips should have a range of 5.5 to 8.0, in 0.2 pH increments. You'll want to test yourself first thing in the morning before eating. Rinse out your mouth, spit on the strip, and then wait for about fifteen seconds. After fifteen seconds, the paper will turn a shade of yellow, blue, or green. A color-coded chart that corresponds to a set of numbers on the pH strip container will tell you whether your pH is acidic or alkaline, and by how much. If you find that you are in the "yellow" (indicating excessive acidity), you'll want to talk to your doctor or nutritionist about changing your diet and adding more alkaline foods, such as veggies, or adding minerals or alkaline water to your diet. By measuring your pH daily or weekly, you'll get a good idea about what foods your body responds well to, and how to keep your pH alkaline.

Foods with Anticancer Properties

We all have unique nutritional requirements, but there are certain categories and types of foods that most of us will respond well to. These are described in the following sections.

"Clean" Animal Protein

By "clean," I mean organic, free-range, hormone- and antibiotic-free animal protein, which is beneficial for most people, and provides essential amino acids and fatty acids that the body needs to heal normal cells and cell membranes. Organic chicken, turkey, and beef; game meat, such as elk, bison, and buffalo; and low-mercury seafood and eggs are some examples of healthy choices of animal protein.

ORGAN MEATS

Organ meats are packed with anticancer properties. Any patient who is weak, tired, and anemic could benefit from consuming grass-fed, organic liver and eating it raw, because liver gives the body energy.

Raw liver doesn't taste that great, though, so you may want to cut it up into very small pieces and swallow the pieces whole, chasing each one down with sips of water. That way, you don't have to taste the liver. I also recommend taking some hydrochloric acid (HCL) beforehand so your stomach can readily break down entire chunks of the liver. If you are severely immune-compromised and/or concerned about eating food raw, taking HCL also ensures that any pathogens that might be present in the meat will be killed off, since one of the functions of HCL is to destroy harmful microbes. If you take HCL, you shouldn't have to worry about microbial contamination from raw liver.[4]

Liver can be stored in the refrigerator or freezer in a little waxed paper bag. Although it might not taste great, all of our patients tell me that it makes them feel better, so chances are, it will make you feel better, too.

Before trying this food in its raw form, consult your doctor to ensure the food is safe for you as an individual to eat.

ORGANIC POULTRY

Free-range organic poultry that hasn't been raised with antibiotics or synthetic hormones is another category of healthy meat. Try some chicken, turkey, quail, and/or duck.

People with cancer often need lots of fat in their diet, so I would recommend leaving the skin on poultry to increase your absorption of its fat content. Avoid breading or battering it, since this increases the carbohydrate content. Otherwise, feel free to prepare it any way that you like: baked, sautéed, broiled, or steamed.

WILD-CAUGHT FISH

Fish can be highly contaminated with mercury and other environmental contaminants, especially larger fish that have a longer life span, as well as farm-raised fish, which are often fed a nonnative diet in unclean environments. Still, fish contains healthy nutrients, such as essential fatty acids (EFAs) that are crucial for maintaining healthy cell membranes, so I recommend eating certain types of fish in moderation.

If you choose to eat fish, select smaller wild-caught fish, such as sardines, haddock, mackerel, and salmon, which tend to be less contaminated with heavy metals than larger fish, such as tuna. I also recommend that you take a heavy metal–binding supplement, such as zeolite or chlorella, whenever you have a meal that contains fish, to mop up any toxins that the fish may release into your body. (I discuss heavy metal binders in greater detail in Chapter 5.) I know this may sound extreme, but we have found that our patients' heavy metal levels increase whenever they eat fish too often. The reality is, much of our food supply is contaminated, so enjoy fish, but don't eat it daily, and always take a heavy metal binder with it.

Finally, it's a good idea to avoid such products as imitation crabmeat, since they sometimes contain added ingredients that some research suggests may be harmful to the body and may also be contaminated with toxins.

ORGANIC EGGS

Eggs are easy to digest and contain high amounts of healthy protein. Always choose free-range eggs from hens that are fed a native diet (not corn) and which are free of growth hormones and antibiotics.

CAREFULLY SOURCED RED MEAT

Red meat, as long as it comes from wild or grass-fed animals that are fed a native diet (that means grass, not corn) and aren't raised with antibiotics or synthetic growth hormones, is healthy for many people. If you are following a ketogenic diet, the more fat that is in the meat, the better because consuming healthy fats encourages your body to use ketones for energy, rather than glucose, which feeds cancer. Red meat also contains essential amino acids, vitamins, and minerals that promote wellness.

That said, too much red meat can create excessive acidity in the body, so it's a good idea to periodically monitor your pH if you eat red meat regularly (three or more times per week). If you find that red meat is contributing to an acidic condition in your body, you can simply reduce your intake of it and replace it with other healthful sources of protein.

If you are a vegetarian or prefer to avoid red meat entirely, you can take a supplemental amino acid product, such as Master Amino Acid Pattern (MAP) or Perfect Amino (the latter of which is more economical than MAP but similar in quality), and make plant-based protein smoothies to ensure your body is getting the protein it needs to repair and regenerate itself. Both of these foods are described later in this chapter.

BONE BROTHS

If you are really sick, you might find that you are frequently cold, and cold people tend to benefit greatly from eating warm foods, such as stews or bone broths. Bone broths are especially good because they contain a number of beneficial elements. For instance, the amino acids in bone broth lower inflammation, as do the broken-down components of cartilage. Bone broths fight infection, and their gelatin helps heal the gut and promote healthy digestion. Further, bone broth contains high amounts of magnesium, calcium, and other nutrients the body needs to function properly and get better. You can purchase delicious ingredients for bone broths online at US Wellness Meats, a company that conducts clean, organic farming. For more information, see the Resources section at the end of this book.

Vegetables

Vegetables are the true foundation of any anticancer diet, especially allium and nonstarchy cruciferous vegetables, which have cancer-prevention properties. *Allium* means "garlic" in Greek; these vegetables include garlic, leeks, shallots, chives, scallions, and yellow and green onions. Studies suggest these veggies may help promote apoptosis, or cancer cell self-destruction. Garlic may be the single most powerful anticancer food because it stimulates the body's immune function. The sulfur compounds found in these foods also reduce the carcinogenic effects of nitrosamines and N-nitroso compounds you may ingest whenever you might overcook or grill meat.

Cruciferous vegetables, such as broccoli, Brussels sprouts, bok choy, Chinese cabbage, cauliflower, kale, and red and curly cabbage, contain the powerful anticancer molecules sulforaphane and indole-3 carbinols (I3Cs). You'll want to avoid boiling your cabbage and broccoli, however, since boiling destroys the sulforaphane and I3Cs. Sauté or steam them instead.

Here is a list of anticancer vegetables:

- Asparagus
- Artichoke
- Bean sprouts
- Beets and beet greens
- Broccoli
- Bok choy
- Brussels sprouts
- Cabbage (red and green)
- Cauliflower
- Celery
- Chinese cabbage
- Chives
- Collard greens
- Cucumber
- Fiddlehead
- Garlic
- Green beans
- Green onions
- Kale
- Leeks
- Lettuce (all kinds)
- Mustard greens
- Parsley
- Radishes
- Rutabaga
- Scallions

- Seaweed, such as kelp and dulse
- Shallots
- Spinach
- Spirulina (an algae)

- Sprouts
- Watercress
- Yellow onions
- Zucchini

If your doctor recommends that you follow a ketogenic diet, you'll want to limit your intake of nightshade vegetables, such as peppers and tomatoes, and completely avoid starchy vegetables, such as carrots, beets, butternut squash, and peas, as these contain higher amounts of carbohydrates. However, these healthy vegetables may be beneficial if you don't do well on a ketogenic or other type of low-carb diet.

Low-Sugar Fruits

Fruit is healthy and beneficial for individuals, barring individuals with food allergies or sensitivities, but when it comes to fighting cancer some fruits do a better job than others. Fruits contain a lot of natural sugar and too much natural sugar can cause an increase in blood sugar levels that stimulates cancer cells to absorb the extra sugar and use it as energy. In general, these are the foods that contain the most anticancer properties, and all of them can be consumed on a ketogenic diet (depending on your carbohydrate threshold):

- Avocados
- Blackberries
- Blueberries
- Boysenberries
- Cranberries

- Lemons
- Limes
- Strawberries
- Raspberries

Nuts, Seeds, and Healthy Fats and Oils

Healthy oils, such as organic olive, hemp, walnut, avocado, and Malaysian red palm and medium-chain triglyceride (MCT) oils, such as palm kernel and coconut oils, are a vital component of any anticancer food plan. They contain essential fatty acids, which your body needs to maintain the integrity of normal cell membranes and reduce inflammation, which is significantly linked to cancer. Cacao butter, both organic and raw, as well as most nuts, such as almonds, walnuts, cashews, and macadamia nuts; seeds; organic mayonnaise; and avocados are additional good sources of healthy fat. I would recommend avoiding peanuts because they may be likely to contain mold and be contaminated with a variety of toxins compared with other kinds of nuts.[5]

If you decide to follow a ketogenic diet, you'll want to consult with your doctor, study a ketogenic diet book, or consult with a nutritionist familiar with the diet to determine how many nuts you can safely eat because nuts contain carbohydrates. Otherwise, they are a great choice of food for most people.

Fresh Herbs and Dried Spices

I encourage you to flavor your food with ample amounts of herbs and spices, such as turmeric, ginger, pepper, cilantro, parsley, rosemary, and oregano to make the most of your dishes and add another anticancer fighting element to your treatment regimen. Many herbs, such as turmeric, have powerful anticancer and anti-inflammatory effects upon the body, so use them liberally in your cooking.

Green, Turmeric, and Ginger Teas

Herbal teas are a great alternative to sodas and sugary drinks, especially green tea, which is loaded with ECGC, one of the most powerful cancer-fighting antioxidants there is. Turmeric and ginger tea are also great for reducing inflammation and contain powerful antioxidants. Ginger, in fact, is a stronger antioxidant than vitamin E! All of these teas can help stimulate apoptosis (cancer cell death), and are thought to inhibit angiogenesis (the creation of new tumor blood vessels). Ginger also helps combat nausea and vomiting, two common side effects of chemotherapy.

Coffee is very acidic, but if you must drink coffee, add some coconut oil to it, which will slow your body's adrenaline response to it and make it more metabolically palatable to your body.

Sweeteners

Stevia is a natural herb that you can use as a substitute for sugar in desserts or to sweeten beverages and smoothies. It is just as sweet as sugar and safe for most people. Unlike sugar, stevia doesn't negatively affect your blood sugar or insulin levels, and doesn't feed fungal infections, which some people with cancer are prone to.

Sea Salt

If you enjoy salt, you can use moderate amounts (500 to 2,000 mg) of unprocessed natural sea salt in your food daily. A single teaspoon of salt provides about 2,000 mg of salt to the body. Himalayan rock salt, Real Salt, or Celtic sea salt are especially beneficial and can help support electrolyte balance in the cells. Cardia Salt is also one of my favorite salts because it contains reduced amounts of sodium but also has essential minerals, such as potassium and magnesium, which the body needs to maintain electrolyte balance and proper cellular function.

Wheatgrass

Wheatgrass is a fantastic anticancer food that provides over forty benefits to the body. It is one of the best sources of chlorophyll, a substance that plants produce when exposed to sunlight. Therefore, it contains more light energy than any other element, and when you consume it, you may find you also get an energy boost. Like all plants that contain chlorophyll, wheatgrass is also high in oxygen. By now you probably know your brain and body function best in a high-oxygen environment, while cancer cells die in such an environment. Chlorophyll also arrests the growth and development of pathogenic bacteria and rebuilds red blood cells in people who are anemic.

And that's just the beginning! Wheatgrass contains over one hundred other elements that benefit the body. For instance, when it is grown in organic soil, it absorbs nearly one hundred minerals from that soil, which makes it a valuable and needed source of minerals. Remember, minerals help keep your body alkaline, which then also helps you fight cancer.

Among its other benefits, wheatgrass can be excellent for detoxification and has proven to be more effective at cleansing the body than carrot juice or any other fruit or vegetable. It can wash drug residue from the body; bind and carry heavy metals out of it; purify the liver; help regulate your blood sugar, blood pressure, circulation and digestion; and increase your strength, endurance, and energy.[6]

Fresh Green Juices

Green vegetable drinks made from such foods as wheatgrass and nonstarchy vegetables provide a highly bioavailable source of nutrients to the body, along with a superdose of enzymes. Among their other benefits, green juices support the mitochondria, those little energy furnaces inside of the cell that give you energy; reduce inflammation; support your immune system; and help eliminate *Candida* and other fungal infections.

In Chapter 13, we share some easy-to-make healthy juicing recipes that promote alkalinity and health. I recommend that you either make your own juice or purchase fresh, unpasteurized juice from a juice bar or other juice vendor. Most juices at your local grocery store are likely to be pasteurized, and pasteurization destroys all of the immune supportive nutrients found in fresh juice. You'll want to make sure to buy unpasteurized juice fresh, though, as bacteria tend to grow in unpasteurized juice that has been on the shelf for more than a couple of days. Many states now have juice bars, where you can buy juice fresh. Alternatively, there are a few companies, such as Suja, that make fresh juice using a process called high-pressure processing (rather than pasteurization), which kills harmful bacteria while preserving all of the healthy nutrients in the juice. You can find this juice at many health food stores nationwide. I recommend high-pressure processed juice for cancer patients.

Protein Smoothies

Your body needs protein to repair tissues and remove toxins, as well as for proper organ function. Protein helps maintain muscle mass, nourish the lining of your gastrointestinal tract, boost your white and red blood cell counts, and heal your tissues. Often, we find that our cancer patients need to increase their intake of protein, especially if they don't consume much meat, have poor digestion, or are showing signs of low muscle density. If this is you, plant protein smoothies are an ideal, delicious way to ensure that you get enough high-quality protein into your diet.

Some clean, healthy plant-based protein products that we recommend can be found in the Resources section. I prefer vegan sources of protein made from hemp, chia, pea, and cranberry, which are suitable for people with casein or lactose sensitivities. You can mix these powders with water or coconut, hemp, or most additive-free nut milks. Avoid protein powders that contain potentially harmful additives or ingredients, such as sugar, soy, or soy protein; maltodextrin, natural flavoring, or any genetically modified or unnatural ingredients.

Pure Water

Your tap water may contain chemical and microbial pollutants that are linked to cancer and other diseases. These contaminants include chlorine, lead, radon (a gas that results from the breakdown of uranium in the ground), parasites, arsenic, chromium, fluoride, uranium, pharmaceutical drug residue, and other harmful chemicals.

If you drink from your tap, consider using an alkalinizing or ionized water filter that not only alkalinizes the water, but also has a solid carbon block filter to remove all chlorine, heavy metals, pharmaceutical drugs, pathogens, industrial chemicals, and other toxins. Many companies, such as Enagic USA and Chanson Water, make these.

If you can't afford these types of filters, which can cost many hundreds or even thousands of dollars, Berkey water filters are a great alternative. They provide many of the same benefits as the more expensive filters and are affordable, at around $200 to $250 for a smaller system. See the Resources section for information about where to purchase these.

Another option is to purchase spring water in glass bottles from your local health food store, or reverse-osmosis or distilled water in 5-gallon bottles. If you really are on a tight budget, you could purchase a Brita water filter, which is sold at retail stores nationwide. These are much less effective at removing contaminants from the water than the other options mentioned here, but they are better than nothing if your resources are limited.

Or, if you can afford it, you might try pHenomenal water, a liquid that you add to distilled water, which causes the water to have a very alkaline pH of about 12.2. Alkaline water neutralizes the harmful acids in your body and helps your body eliminate them, thereby creating an environment that is thought to be less favorable to cancer.

To use pHenomenol water, you need to mix it with distilled water. Distilled water is usually sold in 1-gallon plastic bottles at the grocery store, or you can purchase a distiller for your kitchen faucet so that you can make your own water and avoid the cancer-linked phthalates that leech from plastic bottles into the water. Even BPA-free plastic bottles aren't that safe, so I would recommend either purchasing a filter for your faucet or buying distilled water in glass bottles whenever possible.

In addition to filtered water and tea, another tasty, great anticancer beverage that I suggest is homemade lemonade, which you can make by simply combining sparkling water with lemon and stevia, or by adding a drop of culinary-grade lemon essential oil to filtered or sparkling water.

Master Amino Acid Pattern (MAP) Supplements

Note: You can also substitute a product called Perfect Amino for MAP. However, for the purposes of discussion, we use MAP as an example throughout this chapter, as well as in the Recipes and 14-day plan.

If you don't eat a lot of meat, are vegetarian or vegan, have lost muscle mass due to cancer, or just want to detoxify your body better, we recommend supplementing your diet with a product called Master Amino Acid Pattern (MAP), or Perfect Amino, which is a highly bioavailable amino acid supplement that helps provide your body with all of the amino acids that it needs to repair itself.

Whenever you eat a food, your body will use some of the nutrients in that food to build fatty acids, enzymes, and other proteins or to create energy, but some components of the food will also be excreted as nitrogen and ammonia waste. Cancer patients sometimes have a weak gastrointestinal system and so end up with large amounts of this waste in their body, because they can't effectively digest certain foods, especially animal protein. If this is you, Master Amino Acid Pattern can provide you with the protein you need so you don't have to consume large amounts of animal protein and strain your digestive tract. You can find more information on MAP and dosing guidelines in Chapter 12. For a less-expensive alternative to MAP, you could also try a product called Perfect Amino, which contains all of the same amino acids as MAP, and in the same proportions. See the Resources section for more information.

If you are really sick and can't eat lots of raw foods or animal products, you might try a food plan that consists of steamed nonstarchy vegetables, lots of green juices, and Master Amino Acids, instead of a ketogenic diet or other type of food plan. One advantage of a plant-based diet is that it is also beneficial for your liver and kidneys, and cuts down on the amount of metabolic waste in your body.

A Note About Fasting

Short-term fasting, either in juice or water form, can be beneficial for some individuals. Healthy cells can survive on only small amounts of glucose, whereas cancer cells have greater caloric needs and may be weakened when there is little to no glucose in the body. When you fast, the idea is you help deprive the cancer of the food it needs to survive.

Many studies on fasting show that fasting augments the functioning of the immune system. For example, one study published in 2012 reveals that fasting before chemotherapy treatments improves chemotherapy outcomes.[7] Another study, published in January 2014 in *Cancer and Metastasis Reviews*, shows that radiation treatment outcomes are improved in patients who combine intermittent fasting with a ketogenic diet.[8]

If you decide to fast, it's best to work with a physician who can help you understand the benefits and risks of fasting, and knows whether it would be helpful in your particular case. If you are malnourished, weak, have lost muscle mass, or are severely immune-compromised, you should avoid fasting until you are stronger and healthier.

What *Not* to Eat If You Want to Be Healthy

Now that you know which foods are life giving and beneficial for preventing and fighting cancer, here are a few guidelines about what *not* to eat if you want to keep cancer away.

Inflammatory and Allergenic Foods

No matter what type of food plan you follow, if that plan contains a food that produces an allergic or inflammatory response in your body, you need to avoid it. You can tell when you are allergic to a food because it will usually make you tired or cause you to feel grumpy, brain fogged, or bad in some other way. If you're really not sure, you can ask your integrative doctor to do a food allergy test by using bioenergetic or another type of reliable testing.

If you don't have access to food allergy testing, you could also try doing a food elimination diet. This basically involves omitting a certain food or foods from your diet for a particular amount of time—perhaps a week or two—and observing how you feel after you cut these foods out. If you feel more energetic or happy, or better in some other way, then it is likely you are allergic to one or more of the foods you removed from your diet. To determine which food(s) are the problem, slowly reintroduce each food back into your daily diet, one at a time, and observe how you feel after adding each one. Most people are allergic to what I call the "sensitive seven" and will have an inflammatory response to many or all of the following seven foods, so pay particular attention to how you feel after eating these foods. Or you could simply eliminate them from your diet. They include:

- Dairy products
- Wheat
- Sugar
- Corn
- Soy
- Eggs (Note: Eggs are often okay if they are organic.)
- Peanuts

Also, it goes without saying that you should avoid foods that can be especially toxic in excess, such as alcohol, caffeine, soda, and fast or processed food.

Fried and Grilled Foods

Foods that are fried and grilled can produce cancer-causing compounds in the body that damage DNA. So, don't grill or fry your foods. Instead, bake, sauté, broil, or steam them.

GMO Food

Genetically modified food has been strongly linked to food allergies, leaky gut syndrome, and other health problems. The Environmental Working Group contends that some scientists have observed changes in the metabolism of animals fed GMO food,[9] and many studies have proven that GMO food has adverse effects on the body. For instance, one recent study revealed that lab mice that were fed genetically modified maize developed large mammary tumors more frequently than did mice that were not given GMO maize. They also experienced hormonal disruption, kidney problems, and liver congestion as a result of consuming the food.[10]

While there are many arguments both for and against genetically modifying food, my experience suggests that most people tend to have an allergic or inflammatory reaction to this kind of food. Ultimately, it's best to not let yourself be an experiment, so avoid GMO food as much as possible, and choose organic food instead.

Wheat

Wheat used to be a healthy food, but much of the wheat produced today hardly resembles that which our ancestors ate. Since at least the 1980s, many varieties of wheat have been genetically modified and are no longer prepared and processed according to traditional farming methods. Wheat also contains high amounts of gluten, which has the potential to inflame the gastrointestinal tract and can cause leaky gut syndrome, a condition in which small particles of food "leak" through the intestinal walls into the bloodstream, instead of being digested, and cause inflammation throughout the body. Overly processed wheat also turns to sugar in the body and causes blood sugar spikes that lead to high insulin. Inflammation and high insulin are two major risk factors for cancer, so if you already have cancer, eating wheat that is impure or overly processed is like throwing gasoline on a fire.

Dairy Products

Dairy has become a major food allergy because many dairy products sold in US grocery stores are made from cows that were exposed to antibiotics and hormones. Most farmers routinely administer antibiotics and a growth hormone called recombinant bovine growth hormone (rBGH) to cows, to make them mature faster and keep them infection-free. Cows are susceptible to infections because most are fed corn, which is a mainstay of their diet because it is subsidized by the US government and therefore inexpensive. Unfortunately, cows were not designed to eat corn, so they develop digestive problems and infections from it, which must then be treated with antibiotics. When you consume conventionally raised cow's meat or dairy products, you also consume the antibiotics and growth hormones in these products, which can then cause problems in your body.

Antibiotics, for instance, kill off the beneficial bacteria in your digestive tract, which play an important role in the functioning of your immune system and help kill off pathogenic bacteria. Growth hormones may cause deregulation of your body's own hormones and increase your insulin growth factor-1 (IGF-1) levels. This can dangerous because high IGF-1 levels may foster cancer growth.

Putting It All into Practice

If these guidelines sound stringent, just remember, you must first remodel your body and make sure that you've established order there before you can afford to eat foods that could compromise your health in any way.

When you are ill, you can't cheat on your diet. This is nonnegotiable! We are trying to save your life, so all of your choices matter; what you think, move, say, eat, and drink—all matter. At the end of *The Cancer Revolution,* you'll find simple recipes and meal plans illustrating exactly what kinds of foods you can combine to make great-tasting meals, and how to do so.

I think you will decide that the benefits of eating well and making small sacrifices in your food plan is well worth it, once you see how much better you feel as a result of eliminating the junk from your life.

Whenever my patients get discouraged about having to follow a new diet, I sometimes tell them, "I'm not trying to deprive you of the foods that you like. These are the laws of Mother Nature. I did not make the laws. I'm just trying to get your body to work according to the laws of nature. I'm just the messenger, restoring order to your body." I want you, like my patients, to feel great and live a healthful, happy, long life.

SUMMARY OF ANTICANCER FOODS		
Healthy Anticancer Foods	**Examples**	
Organic meats/animal protein	Organ meats Poultry (chicken, turkey, quail, duck) Small, wild-caught fish (haddock, mackerel, salmon, sardines)	Eggs from free-range chicken Lean red meat (from bison, buffalo, elk, deer, lamb, cow) Bone broths
Organic green and nonstarchy vegetables	Asparagus Artichokes Bean sprouts Beets Broccoli Bok choy Brussels sprouts Cabbage Cauliflower Celery Chinese cabbage Chives Collard greens Cucumbers Fiddleheads Garlic Green beans Green onions	Kale Leeks Lettuce (all kinds) Mustard greens Onions Parsley Radishes Red and curly cabbage Rutabaga Scallions Sea vegetables, such as organic kelp, dulse, and spirulina Shallots Spinach Sprouts Watercress Yellow and green onions Zucchini

continues

SUMMARY OF ANTICANCER FOODS

Healthy Anticancer Foods	Examples	
Organic nightshades, higher-glycemic, and starchy vegetables (for some people only)	Beets Bell peppers Eggplant Mushrooms Parsnips Red potatoes	Squash (all kinds) Sweet potatoes Tomatoes Yams Yucca
Organic low-glycemic fruit	Avocados Blackberries Blueberries Boysenberries	Lemons Limes Raspberries Strawberries
Organic nuts and seeds	Almonds Cashews Macadamia nuts Pumpkin seeds	Sesame seeds Sunflower seeds Walnuts
Healthy fats and oils	Cacao butter Coconut oil Hemp seed oil	Malaysian red palm oil MCT oil Olive oil
Fresh herbs and spices	Cilantro Garlic Ginger Oregano	Parsley Pepper Rosemary Turmeric
Herbal teas	Ginger Green	Turmeric
Wheatgrass		
Stevia		
Sea salt		
Fresh green juices	See Chapter 13.	
Plant protein powder (for smoothies)	Chia seed Cranberry	Hemp seed Pea
Pure water		
Dairy	Goat cheese (raw)	Goat's milk yogurt (raw)

SUSAN'S Story

I was diagnosed with a stage 2A breast cancer and initially had a lumpectomy to remove it, along with radiation treatments. I then found Dr. Connealy and continued my healing regimen through the Cancer Center for Healing because I believed I needed tools beyond what conventional medicine had to offer. And, sure enough, thermography screening revealed I still had cancer.

I had already done a lot of research and learned about the importance of diet in healing. As a result of my research, I got a really clear understanding about how diet affects the hormones and healing from cancer.

So, when I showed up at Dr. Connealy's door, I was already armed with a lot of knowledge and was thrilled to discover that we were on the same page. In contrast, nobody at the cancer center where I had received radiation treatments had any notion about what a cancer diet should look like. They had no opinion on sugar; instead, they said, "Eat ice cream; make yourself feel better."

As part of my healing process, I went on a ketogenic diet, which made me feel great. It really agreed with me, and I found my weight easy to control while on it. It helped me lose unnecessary fat, which I believe also contributed to my healing.

After a couple of years of working with Dr. Connealy, I am now cancer-free. Many different treatments helped me get better, but I feel that being on the right diet was the most important aspect of my regimen because it was something I could control and it made sense to me.

CHAPTER 5

Remove Toxins to Boost Your Health

> ## IN THIS CHAPTER, YOU WILL LEARN . . .
>
> - What environmental toxins are linked to cancer and why
> - How your body's seven detoxification channels function
> - Tools and therapies for eliminating toxins from your body

Whether we like it or not, we are living in a sea of chemicals. There are many thousands of toxic chemicals in the environment, and that number is growing by the day. Nevertheless, only a fraction of these chemicals are tested for their potentially toxic effects upon the body. Consequently, the number of people being diagnosed with autoimmune disorders, cancer, and other severe, chronic degenerative diseases is increasing, which suggests these toxins are negatively affecting our health.

We all need to take a look around and get proactive about removing toxins that could be making us more susceptible to cancer and other illnesses. We can't turn the world around overnight, but we can change our immediate environment and enhance our body's natural detoxification systems to help prevent any potential damage these contaminants may impose.

In this chapter, you'll learn about some of the toxins that research links to cancer, as well as how to safely remove them from your body. Many of the strategies that I describe are simple things that you can do at home. For

75

others, you'll want to enlist the help of a qualified integrative naturopath, medical doctor, or other health-care practitioner experienced in detoxification. You can find a doctor experienced in integrative cancer treatment and detoxification at integrative medical associations, such as the Academy for Comprehensive Integrative Medicine, the American College for Advancement in Medicine, and the International Organization of Integrative Cancer Physicians. See the Resources section at the end of this book for more information.

Types of Cancer-Causing Toxins

In Chapter 1, I briefly mentioned some common sources of toxins that are associated with cancer. The following is an overview of some of the most important of these.

Heavy Metals

Heavy metal toxins, such as mercury, lead, cadmium, and aluminum, are among the most damaging cancer-linked toxins to which we are all exposed. Mercury, which is the second-most-toxic substance in the world, can be found in the air, as well as our food, water supply, personal care products, and our dental amalgams, which is a mixture commonly used in fillings. Metals are even present in less obvious sources, such as cosmetics. For instance, one 2014 study of thirty different types of lipstick used by women in China showed *all* brands of lipstick to contain lead![1] And aluminum is found in nearly all antiperspirants.

In Chapter 11, I describe how to find household and personal care products that are free of potentially harmful metals and other toxic chemicals. After you do this, you'll then want to get the metals removed from your body, with the help of a qualified health-care practitioner, since (unlike most types of detoxification therapy described in this chapter), heavy metal removal isn't a do-it-yourself process. You can find a doctor in your area who does heavy metal removal by doing a search on the medical association websites noted in the previous section. Most good integrative doctors are at least familiar with heavy metal detoxification and can direct you to a resource where you can get help with this. Be sure to consult your oncologist before taking this step.

Pesticides

Pesticides are chemical substances that are used to kill or repel insects, certain plants, and/or animals—not only can they be toxic to those plants and animals, but they are also capable of posing a toxic threat to us. They are sprayed on most conventional produce, so when you eat that produce, you also ingest those chemicals. According to the Pesticide Action Network (PAN), an organization dedicated to educating and finding alternative solutions to the use of hazardous pesticides, "Chemicals can trigger cancer in a variety of ways, including by disrupting hormones, damaging DNA, inflaming tissues and turning genes on or off. Many pesticides are known to cause cancer, and (as the Panel notes) everyone in the United States is exposed to them on a daily basis."[2]

PAN warns, "Children are at a particularly high risk of developing cancer from pesticides as their bodies develop. . . . When parents are exposed to pesticides before a child is conceived, that child's risk of cancer goes up. Pesticide exposures during pregnancy and throughout childhood also increase the risk of childhood cancer."[3]

Plastics

Plastics may be the biggest pollutant in our environment today. So many things contain plastics, from our water bottles and food storage containers, to the wrap that's used to package our cheese and bread, and basically everything that we buy. But like heavy metals, plastics are also found in less obvious places, such as our cars and furniture, which outgas it into the air. So, we don't just ingest plastics but also inhale them.

Also, like heavy metals, plastics have the potential to harm the body in various ways. For instance, they may deactivate and damage peroxisomes, which are little structures inside of the cell that help you detoxify. When your peroxisomes are damaged, greater amounts of toxins can build up inside your body because the cellular structures that are involved in detoxification are broken.

Plastics are xenoestrogens, which, if you'll recall from Chapter 2, are chemicals and toxins that have estrogen-like effects on the body. Natural estrogen is good for us, but xenoestrogens are associated with cancer because they have the potential to disrupt proper hormonal balance.

In Chapter 11, I describe some common household sources of plastic and how to remove them from your environment. Plastics are very difficult to remove from the body with toxin binders, but the good news is that you *can* eliminate them, with an infrared sauna. Later in this chapter I describe infrared sauna therapy and why it's such a great method from removing all kinds of toxins.

Polluted Water

As mentioned, tap water has the potential to contain contaminants that may increase your risk of cancer. I have already recommended a few things that you can do to clean up your drinking water, such as purchasing a filter or filtration system for your faucet or sink. But you'll also want to detoxify your body from any pollutants resulting from previous exposure to bad water. The therapies in this chapter will help you do that.

Immunosuppressant Drugs

Sometimes, taking medication is appropriate and necessary, but medication has the potential to interfere with your body's magnificent biochemistry, and cause some side effect or complication. You can check this out for yourself by consulting the *Physician's Desk Reference*, which lists all types of medications and their side effects.

It's better to find an integrative doctor who can help you find natural alternatives to medications whenever possible and help you correct the underlying cause of disease, instead of just masking your symptoms with drugs.

Dental Toxins

People often view problems in the mouth as if they only affected the mouth, but isn't your mouth connected to the rest of your body? Mine was, the last time I looked! Many of us have weakened organs and a compromised immune system as a result of problems in our mouth. For instance, dental amalgams contain methyl-mercury, a dangerous metal that is believed by many integrative doctors and biological dentists to outgas tiny particles of metal into your brain and the rest of your body every time that you chew. You may also have hidden infections in your mouth caused by root canals or wisdom tooth extractions.

Your mouth needs to be clean and clear of infections and toxins if you want to get well, so if you have infections in your mouth or dental amalgams, you should get them removed by a biological dentist, who will typically understand the dangers of these things and how to safely remove or eliminate them. You can get a referral for a good biological dentist from an organization called Huggins Applied Healing or the International Academy of Oral Medicine and Toxicology, which are dedicated to promoting public health and research-based safe dental procedures. See the Resources section for information about how to contact these organizations.

Electromagnetic Pollution

We are all immersed in a sea of electromagnetic smog daily, which comes from the combined electromagnetic fields (EMFs) emitted by power lines, appliances, computers, cell phones, Wi-Fi, smart meters, and microwave towers—just to name a few sources! While technology has in some ways made our lives easier, we are now being faced with potentially harmful electro-pollution, which was basically unheard of a century ago. Thomas Edison did a good thing by inventing the lightbulb around a century ago, but back then, only 1 in 100 people were diagnosed with cancer.

Too much exposure to electromagnetic fields causes the cells to vibrate, and more rapidly divide and mutate. EMFs are so dangerous that some experts, such as the late Robert O. Becker, MD, an orthopedic surgeon and electro-medicine researcher known as the "father of electromedicine," have called electromagnetic pollution the greatest danger to humanity today.[4]

You're probably not going to get rid of your cell phone, iPad, or computer after you read this, and it wouldn't be realistic for you to do that anyway, but I would advise taking measures to reduce your exposure to the dangerous fields that these gadgets and other sources of EMFs have the potential to generate.

For instance, it's a good idea to keep your cell phone in "airplane" mode or at least away from your body when you aren't using it, and when you are talking, use it only in "speaker phone" mode. If you have a laptop, use it on battery power, rather than plugged into the wall, and use a hard-wired Internet connection whenever you can, rather than Wi-Fi. When you sleep at night, turn off all the electrical appliances in your bedroom, or better yet, turn off all the circuit breakers in your home.

Additionally, a practice that I've found useful is grounding, which involves connecting your body with the earth, either by walking barefoot outside, or contacting your skin with what are called "grounding mats" or "grounding sheets," which you sleep or place your feet on. The mats and sheets connect your body to the earth through your electrical outlets. Grounding may be beneficial because there are natural energetic frequencies within the earth that help balance your body's natural energy and reduce the negative effects of harmful energies from the environment. So, I'd recommend taking a walk barefooted daily; in the grass, dirt, or on the beach (if you live near one). Or get a grounding mat to rest your feet on during the day while you work at the computer, or some grounding sheets to help you rejuvenate and sleep better at night.

Alternatively, you can purchase devices that will partially block the effects of EMFs in your home. For example, Graham-Stetzer filters plug into your electrical outlets and lower the EMFs that are emitted from your smart meter or electrical wiring. It is beyond the scope of this book to describe every type of EMF-protective device, so I would recommend checking out different EMF products, which are available at a variety of online retailers. See the Resources section for more information, including where to purchase EMF-protective devices. You can also learn more about EMF pollution through Kerry Crofton's *A Wellness Guide for the Digital Age: With Safer-Tech Solutions for All Things Wired & Wireless—For Brains Worth Saving.*

"Sick Building" Syndrome

"Sick building syndrome" describes buildings that contain potentially toxic pollutants, such as mold, radon, lead-based paint, and formaldehyde-containing carpet. Water-damaged, new, and/or renovated buildings often have high amounts of these contaminants. If you live or work in a sick building, you should either have that building remediated or consider moving, as your immune system will have a harder time recovering from cancer if you you're exposed to mold and potentially toxic chemicals. Building biologists can often fix some of the problems associated with sick building syndrome. The International Institute for Building Biology and Ecology can refer you to building biologists in the United States who can help. See the Resources section for more information. In Chapter 11, I describe some things you can do to remove toxins from your home in the meantime.

Ionizing and Nuclear Radiation

Ionizing radiation comes from imaging tests, such as chest X-rays, and CT and PET scans, as well as from radiation that gets released from nuclear power plant accidents, such as the Fukushima Daiichi accident that happened in 2011 in Japan. This type of radiation causes DNA damage and cellular mutations that can lead to cancer, so you'll want to avoid unnecessary imaging tests and stay away from areas where nuclear accidents have occurred. Some supplements, such as zeolite and iodine, can help bind with the toxic radioactive elements in your body and carry them out. Zeolite is described later in this chapter.

Infections

Many of us have stealth bacterial, parasitic, viral, and fungal infections, which are passed on into our body from the food, water, and air supply. They drag our immune system down and cause inflammation, which makes it harder for us to prevent or battle cancer.

As I mentioned in Chapter 1, research suggests some infections may also directly cause cancer. For instance, fungal infections have been linked to a whole range of diseases, including cancer. It's fairly easy to get a fungus; for instance, if you take antibiotics or birth control pills or eat excess amounts of sugar, you may increase your risk for candidiasis, which is a type of fungal infection known commonly as thrush or a yeast infection.

Parasitic infections are also easy to contract, and many parasites have been linked to specific types of cancer. Just because you live in the United States or another industrialized nation doesn't mean that you couldn't possibly get sick from parasites. Many hundreds of species of parasites exist, and many of us are infected with some of these, but we don't realize it. If you have a parasite infection, sometimes you will have symptoms but not always. Unfortunately, there is no adequate parasite stool test for detecting parasites because for the test to be effective, the stool must be examined within twenty minutes of a bowel movement, and that's not always possible.

Many studies also substantiate a very strong connection between certain viruses and specific types of cancer. For instance, as I mentioned in Chapter 1, the human papilloma virus (HPV) has been associated with head and neck cancers as well as cervical cancer. Epstein-Barr virus (EBV) has been found in many people with leukemia, and hepatitis C has been linked to liver cancer. Herpes II increases cancer risk in general.

You can find out whether you have stealth infections in your body by checking your blood or by asking your integrative doctor to do a bioenergetic test with a device, such as the ZYTO. Many integrative and naturopathic doctors now use this type of testing.

Most integrative doctors use a wide variety of herbal and pharmaceutical remedies to treat infections. If you have stealth infections in your body, it's important to treat them because they can compromise your recovery from cancer or may set up conditions in your body that are favorable to its development.

Other Environmental Toxins

Because there are literally thousands of toxins in the environment, it is beyond the scope of this book to describe all of them, but by now you should have a pretty good idea about the major types of cancer-causing pollutants that are out there and how to reduce their effects upon your environment. Chapter 1 briefly lists additional sources of toxins that you may want to research on your own. In the meantime, in the following sections, I will share some detoxification strategies that you can do yourself at home to remove these toxins, as well as a few practitioner-assisted strategies.

Detoxification Therapies

Our body removes toxins via seven primary channels: the bowels, the blood, the skin, the kidneys, the lymphatic system, the lungs, and the liver. The detoxification strategies I recommend in the following sections are meant to aid all of these channels, and aim to make the most of your detoxification regimen, and avoid overloading any one organ or system. You can do many of these therapies yourself at home with clearance from your oncologist. For others, you'll want to enlist direct assistance from a qualified integrative doctor or other health-care practitioner experienced in toxin removal.

Lymphatic Drainage Therapies

The most underrated system in your body is your lymphatic system, which is a type of circulatory system that is also part of your waste elimination system. Your body really has two circulatory systems: the blood system and the lymphatic system. Your blood delivers the "groceries," or the nutrients to your cells, while your lymph removes the "garbage," or toxins.

Lymph is a clear fluid that shuttles disease-fighting agents to your cells while transporting dead germs away via a network of lymphatic channels that run throughout your body. These channels comprise the primary transportation system that immune cells, such as macrophages, T-cells, B-cells, and lymphocytes, use to get to the cancer, viruses, fungi, and bacteria. The system also contains over six hundred waste collection sites called lymph nodes, where toxins tend to accumulate. However, unlike your blood, which is pumped and moved through your circulatory system by your heart, your lymphatic system doesn't have any kind of automatic valve system to activate the movement of lymph, which means that this system often gets blocked and the lymph flow, stagnant.

When this happens, your cancer and infection-fighting immune cells can get stuck in the fluid and can't get to their final destination in the cells. You then become defenseless against attacks by viruses, fungi, bacteria, and cancer. Without proper lymphatic flow, germs grow, your blood loses necessary protein, your immune system falters, and infectious diseases march in.

Most blockages within the lymphatic system occur at the lymph nodes. The largest lymph nodes are found primarily around your armpits, just below your jawbone, or in the crease between your thigh and pelvic area. You can sometimes feel your lymph nodes by pressing on and around these areas. At times, you may feel small bumps or even pain. The bumps and pain may indicate blocked lymph nodes or a breakdown in the functioning of the lymphatic system.

Despite the importance of the lymphatic system, some health-care practitioners may never consider the critical role it plays in helping the body fight cancer, but if you want to arm yourself as best you can against the disease, you must make sure that this system is functioning properly. There are many different theories thought to help drain the lymphatic system; here are a few that stand out.

Dry skin brushing. This is a great do-it-yourself technique that may help stimulate lymph flow. For this, you take a long-handled, soft, natural-fiber brush, which you can purchase at your local health food store, and brush your skin in long, broad strokes toward the direction of your heart. You'll want to brush both sides of your body, including your arms, legs, abdomen, chest, back, hands, and feet. The brushing movement stimulates lymphatic flow and breaks up blockages in the lymphatic system. It feels a little prickly at first, but over time, your skin gets used to it. It's recommended that dry skin brushing be done for just five to ten minutes daily.

Rebounding. This is another easy at-home therapy, which simply involves bouncing up and down gently on a mini-trampoline or a large rubber ball for about ten minutes daily. This may help stimulate the flow of lymph and also breaks up blockages in the lymph nodes.

Manual lymph drainage. If you have more resources, you could see a massage therapist or other health-care practitioner that does manual lymph drainage which is a gentle, light-touch, bodywork technique that's designed to stimulate the lymphatic system, drain stagnant fluids, reduce edema, encourage relaxation and stress reduction, and improve sleep. Many massage therapists know how to do this, so ask around to find one in your area who can help you.

Oil Pulling

Oil pulling, an ancient practice with roots in Ayurvedic healing, is a simple, inexpensive technique that you can do at home. For this, you simply swish a healthy type of oil (e.g., coconut or olive oil) around in your mouth, for about five minutes, and then spit it into the sink. The oil binds with the toxins in your mouth and bloodstream.

Some people recommend doing oil pulling for twenty minutes daily for best results, but if you don't have twenty minutes to spare during the day, you can get decent results after about five minutes. Just remember to not swallow the oil while swishing it around in your mouth, or you will also swallow the chemicals and toxins that have been bound up in the oil! And make sure that the oil you use is organic.

Epsom Salt Baths

Epsom salt baths are another simple, inexpensive way to cleanse your body of waste from the comfort of your home. Epsom salt is a pure mineral compound that contains magnesium and sulfate. The magnesium in Epsom salt can help your body function in a number of ways. Magnesium is responsible for regulating the activity of over 324 enzymes, reducing inflammation and aiding in muscle and nerve function, among other important tasks. Sulfates help improve the absorption of nutrients and flush toxins from the body. We often recommend Epsom salt baths to our patients for their detoxification, nutritional, and pain-relieving benefits. Simply pour a cup of Epsom salt under running water into the tub and then soak there for twenty minutes. Warm or hot baths work best.

Castor Oil Pack Therapy

One gentle way you can remove toxins from your liver is with a castor oil pack. Castor oil has been used as a healing agent for centuries; heat combines with the castor oil to help increase blood circulation to your liver and pull toxins out of it through your skin. This is an easy and painless way to aid in keeping your liver clean and functioning well, so it can more easily remove toxins that are associated with cancer. For this therapy, you'll need:

- Castor oil (You may want do a patch test first on your skin to make sure you aren't allergic to the oil—or, even better, ask your doctor to test you for the allergy before trying this therapy)
- 8 x 10-inch cotton flannel cloth
- Hot water bottle or heating pad
- Piece of heavy plastic or a plastic bag that is slightly larger than the flannel cloth (to separate the heating pad from the oiled cloth so you don't get the heating pad dirty)

Once you have all of your materials, you'll want to do the following:

1. Fill a hot water bottle with hot (but not boiling) water.
2. Apply a few tablespoons of castor oil to the flannel cloth and spread it evenly around the cloth until it is fully saturated with oil.
3. Lie down on a bed or sofa, and place the cloth over your liver (which is located on the right side of your abdomen, right under your rib cage).
4. Cover the flannel cloth with the plastic bag, and place the hot water bottle or heating pad on top of the plastic. The plastic helps keep the bag clean and oil-free.
5. Apply heat to the area for thirty to sixty minutes.
6. When the time is up, clean your skin with some water and baking soda. You can store the oily cloth in a plastic bag in the refrigerator for future use.

Juicing

Juicing green vegetables or blending veggies in a blender or Vitamix is another great way thought to help improve the body's natural detoxification system. In Chapter 13, we describe some fantastic juicing recipes that can work well for this purpose. Juicing is especially great if you are weak and can't handle some of the more intense therapies described in this chapter.

Physician-Guided Detox Therapies

Note: The rest of the therapies in this chapter are best done under direct physician supervision. Two of the principal therapies described here—namely, coffee enemas and liver flush cleanses—are fantastic for cleansing the body, but you should not do them if you have been diagnosed with gallbladder problems; significant hemorrhoids, rectal fissures or other rectal problems, or severe mineral deficiencies, unless your doctor recommends them. You should also not do them if you have abdominal pain or gastroenteritis, or if you have had a recent surgery on your colon. If you have been diagnosed as having large gallstones, ask your doctor to help you first dissolve the gallstones before doing the liver flush cleanse and/or coffee enema. There are safe methods for doing this. Once the gallstones have been dissolved, you may be able to do the therapies.

If you are weak or have cachexia (muscle wasting), you should also not do coffee enemas or liver flushes until you are stronger, unless your doctor recommends them. If you are weak, I recommend doing juicing, oil pulling, Epsom salt baths, and/or lymphatic drainage as your primary detoxification-aiding therapies. Then, once your health condition has stabilized and/or you become stronger, you can add the therapies described in the following sections to your regimen.

Coffee Enemas

One of the most important detox therapies are coffee enemas, which can be a powerful way to reduce toxins in your body—up to 700 percent, by some estimates.[5] If you are truly serious about transforming your health in dramatic ways, implementing coffee enemas into your daily routine can bring about life-changing results. Coffee, when taken as an enema, goes preferentially into the liver, and does not enter the body's circulatory system, unless the enema is performed improperly. Therefore, the caffeine in the coffee used for enemas shouldn't stimulate your nervous system or otherwise adversely affect your body, unlike when you drink it. Nonetheless, you may prefer to do enemas in the morning, rather than the evening, in the event a small amount of coffee escapes from the colon into the circulatory system—an effect that can cause overstimulation and prevent you from falling asleep.

Coffee enemas have been around for one hundred years. They were first discovered by a group of WWI nurses who were aiding wounded military soldiers. Since then, research has further suggested their effectiveness for reducing symptoms of toxicity. They are thought to help cleanse and strengthen the body, but for them to work properly, you have to use a certain type of coffee—not the kind you buy at your regular coffee shop! According to the late Max Gerson, a German medical doctor and pioneer of coffee enema therapy, and the famous Gerson diet for cancer patients, caffeine and other beneficial compounds in coffee enemas stimulate the production of glutathione S-transferase (GST) in the liver.[6] GST is an enzyme thought to be your body's "master detoxifier" because it binds with toxins throughout your body and flushes them out during the enema process.

Among their many other benefits, coffee enemas may:

- Improve bile flow and prevent the reabsorption of bile and the toxins contained in expelled bile back into the body. Bile is a dark green to yellowish brown fluid that is produced by the liver that aids in fat digestion.
- Increase the activity and efficiency of protective enzyme systems in your liver and gut that bind toxins so these toxins can be safely eliminated
- Cleanse the colon and digestive tract, and improve the movement of food through the digestive tract. By regularly taking coffee enemas, you can help keep your digestive tract clean, and free of debris and toxic buildup.
- Relieve chronic pain and ease symptoms that may result from detoxification and eliminating too many toxins all at once
- Boost your energy levels, and improve your mental clarity and mood
- Detoxify and enhance your liver

Liver Flush Cleanse

A liver flush cleanse is another powerful therapy thought to help cleanse your liver and gallbladder of toxins, and improve your body's detoxification functions. Many of us have gallstones, which build up in our liver and gallbladder over time, and compromise the function of these organs. Gallstones are made from cholesterol, bilirubin, and other components of bile, and can be as small as a grain of sand, or as large as a golf ball. Many diseases have been linked to gallstones, so you can do a lot for your health by periodically eliminating these stones.

The following is a liver flush cleanse that you can do at home. As noted earlier in this chapter, it is best to consult with your physician before doing the cleanse.

Liver Flush Cleanse Ingredients
- 3 tablespoons of Epsom salt (Epsom salt is usually sold in a pint- or quart-size carton or bag. You can use the remainder of the salt for baths.)
- 2 teaspoons of Vitality C or another brand of high-potency liquid or powdered vitamin C (4,000 mg per teaspoon)
- 10 drops of freshly squeezed, organic lemon juice (optional)
- 4 (500 mg) capsules of L-ornithine. This can be purchased at your local health food store or at a variety of online retailers.
- 1 cup of olive oil
- 1 large or 2 small freshly squeezed whole organic pink grapefruit

Preparation

First, you'll want to do the liver cleanse on a day when you will be able to take the following morning off from eating immediately as well as from any daily responsibilities, such as work. Eat a low-fat breakfast and lunch the day that you begin.

The Day of the Cleanse

2:00 p.m.: Do not eat or drink anything after 2:00 p.m. Sipping water is okay if you get thirsty.

6:00 p.m.: Mix together 1 tablespoon of Epsom salt and 1 teaspoon of Vitality C in a cup of cold water. You may also add 10 drops of freshly squeezed organic lemon juice to improve the taste, if you wish. You may also want to take a few swallows of water afterward to rinse your mouth.

8:00 p.m.: Repeat the procedure and drink the same solution that you did at 6:00 p.m.

9:45 p.m.: Mix 4 (500 mg) capsules of L-ornithine capsules, along with 1 cup of olive oil and 1 cup of freshly squeezed grapefruit juice, in a glass jar. Shake the mixture and then drink it.

10:00 p.m.: After your 9:45 p.m. drink, lie down flat. Do not stay up and do anything; go straight to bed.

Next Morning

Upon awakening, mix 1 tablespoon of Epsom salt with 1 teaspoon of Vitality C in a cup of cold water, and drink the mixture anytime after 6:00 a.m. (You can go back to bed after this if you wish.)

Two hours after awakening: Drink another cup of water with Epsom salt and Vitality C (using the same amounts described above).

Two hours later, you may eat food. Start with your favorite fruit. When you feel hungry, eat a light lunch, and by suppertime you should be able to eat a normal meal.

What to Expect During the Liver Flush

The morning after the flush, expect your stools to be watery and to contain green and brown pea-size stones. Sometimes the bile ducts are full of cholesterol crystals that have not yet formed into stones. They appear as chaff, which are shiny crystals that float on the top of the water. Cleansing chaff is just as important as purging stones.

You'll want to do this cleanse periodically; as often as every two weeks, if you wish, until your liver is free of any stones or chaff. Then, once your liver is no longer expelling stones or other debris, do the liver cleanse twice yearly for continued health maintenance. As I mentioned earlier, liver flushes can be inadvisable for people with some health conditions and taxing on the body. For instance, some people may experience mild nausea or abdominal pain after drinking the olive oil solution, or feel a little tired for several days afterward, so it's best to consult with your doctor before doing one, to make sure that it's beneficial and safe for you.

Infrared Sauna Therapy

Your skin is your body's largest detoxification organ, and it plays a major role in removing toxins from your body. Sauna therapy is one great way to make use of this organ because it causes you to eliminate toxins through your sweat, and has been recognized throughout history as a powerful way to relax, cleanse your body, and improve your overall health. It uses radiant, infrared energy to help mobilize toxins from deep within your tissues, as it rejuvenates your body.

Sauna therapy cleanses and detoxifies your body of difficult-to-remove toxins, such as pesticides, PCBs, drug residues, acidic wastes, and heavy metals. It also helps improve your circulation, bring oxygen to your tissues, and enhance nutrient delivery to your cells. It stimulates your immune system and improves your cardiovascular (heart) and pulmonary (lung) function, and helps resolve inflammation and edema.

It is also a great way to release stress in a comfortable, warm environment! Japanese researchers have also reported that infrared radiant heat antidotes may nullify the negative effects of toxic electromagnetic pollution upon the body.[7]

Not all saunas are created equal. The energy of infrared saunas may be two or three times that of a hot air sauna, which is the type of sauna that you'd typically find at your local gym, yet they operate within a significantly cooler air temperature range of 110° to 130°F. Compare this to hot air saunas, which operate at temperatures of 180° to 235°F. The lower heat range of infrared saunas is thought to be safer and more comfortable for people who have cardiovascular and other health problems.

I've been using an infrared sauna almost daily for five years. I usually do a sauna session between seeing my morning and afternoon patients, and it's invigorating. You can do sauna therapy at some medical clinics, spas, or even at a gym (if you can't afford to go to a clinic), or you can purchase your own sauna for at-home use. New and used two-person saunas range in price from $800 to $3,000, although you can also purchase portable fabric sauna tents for $100 to $200. While possibly not as effective as a full infrared sauna, they can nonetheless provide you with some of the same benefits by causing you to sweat. See the Resources section at the end of this book for more information on where to purchase saunas.

Sauna therapy is generally safe for everyone, but as with some of the other detox strategies in this chapter, it's always best to consult with your doctor before doing it, to make sure that you don't have a health condition for which it is contraindicated. For instance, some people with unstable hypertension (high blood pressure) or very low blood pressure (hypotension) may not be able to do sauna therapy.

Colonic Irrigation/Hydrotherapy

Colonic irrigation or hydrotherapy, sometimes called a "colonic," involves flushing and cleansing the colon with warm filtered water. Colonics are thought to help remove waste and toxins that build up in the colon, and that may promote the growth of cancer cells. Essentially, they flush away fecal matter that may be left over after regular bowel movements and could interfere with your body's ability to absorb nutrients. They may be especially beneficial if you have a large tumor because tumors can break up and cause necrotic areas (areas of dead tissue) in the body. The body expels these toxic byproducts through the colon, so colonic irrigation can help your body eliminate these toxins more effectively and rapidly.

Colonic irrigation has other benefits. Among these, it can improve your circulation, immune function and appetite; eliminate headaches, and boost your energy. It is a great way to eliminate toxins, whether or not you have cancer. Colonic irrigation isn't a do-it-yourself therapy, however. To find a colonic irrigation practitioner in your area, simply do an Internet search, and keyboard the term "colon hydrotherapy," along with your local town or city name, into the search box.

Other Detoxification Therapies

EDTA Chelation Therapy

Chelation therapy is used to remove heavy metals from the body and has been around for fifty years. Integrative doctors often do heavy metal testing on patients and sometimes recommend chelation as part of their recovery plan because metals may interfere with many chemical reactions in the body and could paralyze the cells, thus compromising an individual's cancer battle.

One of the best chelating agents that doctors who are well versed in detoxification will use on their patients is ethylene-diamine-tetra-acetic acid (EDTA), which is a synthetic amino acid related to vinegar that binds with toxins and carries them from the body, especially heavy metals, such as lead. A study published in the *Journal of Advancement in Medicine* found a 90 percent reduction in mortality in fifty-nine cancer patients who took EDTA during their eighteen years of follow-up treatment.[8]

EDTA can be taken orally or intravenously. However, heavy metal chelation, unlike some of the other detoxification methods discussed in this chapter, should absolutely only be done under physician supervision, as heavy metal removal is an art, and mistakes in dosing can cause serious problems, including redistribution of metals to other parts of the body. So, you'll want to make sure to find a doctor who understands heavy metal detoxification by doing a search or asking for a referral from one of the medical association websites listed in the Resources.

Toxin-Binding Agents

Another way you can help remove toxins from your body is by taking toxin-binding supplements or agents. These are natural nutritional or chemical substances that bind with and carry toxins out of the body. For instance, zeolite and chlorella are two all-around great binders that we recommend to our patients that will "vacuum-clean" all kinds of toxins from the body. See the Resources section for specific dosing and product recommendations.

Detox for Life

If you choose only one health tool to aid in your cancer fight, make it detoxification therapy. After doing some of these therapies, you are likely to find you will have more energy, less pain, a clearer mind, better sleep, and/or a reduction in other symptoms. If you are wondering which of these therapies you should do and when, Chapter 12 offers a sample 14-day plan for incorporating some of them into your daily life. Or you can consult with an experienced integrative cancer and detox specialist, who will help customize a plan for you. By making detoxification a daily part of your life, you will help arm and equip yourself to not only more effectively prevent cancer and other diseases, but you also will feel stronger and healthier as you cope with and fight whatever ails you.

SUMMARY CHART OF DETOX THERAPIES

Detoxification Therapies	Primary Benefits
Lymphatic drainage (dry body brushing, rebounding, manual lymph drainage) Can be done at home, except for manual lymph drainage, which requires professional assistance	• Breaks up stagnant lymph fluid so that disease-fighting agents can more easily get to the cells and dead germs can be more effectively eliminated
Oil pulling Can be done at home	• Removes toxins that are circulating in the bloodstream and mouth
Epsom salt bath Can be done at home	• Pulls toxins out of the body through the skin • Relaxes the muscles • Improves blood flow
Castor oil pack Can be done at home	• Pulls toxins out of the liver through the skin
Juicing	• See Chapter 13.
Coffee enema Can be done at home but doctor supervision is highly recommended	• Improves bile flow • Increases the activity and efficiency of protective enzyme systems in the liver and gut that bind toxins • Cleanses and heals the liver, colon, and digestive tract • Improves the movement of food through the digestive tract • Relieves chronic pain and eases symptoms that result from detoxification • Boosts energy levels and improves mental clarity and mood • Detoxifies and repairs the liver
Liver flush cleanse	• Cleanses and heals the liver, gallbladder, colon, and digestive tract • Removes gallstones • Relieves chronic pain and eases symptoms that result from detoxification • Boosts energy levels and improves mental clarity and mood
Infrared sauna Can be done at home or at a clinic	• Cleanses and detoxifies the body of difficult-to-remove toxins, such as pesticides, PCBs, drug residues, acidic wastes, and heavy metals • Improves circulation • Brings oxygen to the tissues • Improves nutrient delivery to the cells • Stimulates immune system function • Improves cardiovascular (heart) and pulmonary (lung) function • Helps resolve inflammation and edema • Helps release stress
Colonic irrigation/hydrotherapy Requires a professional	• Eliminates fecal matter buildup in colon • Improves circulation • Stimulates immune function and appetite • Eliminates headaches and boosts energy.

continues

SUMMARY CHART OF DETOX THERAPIES   continued

Detoxification Therapies	Primary Benefits
IV EDTA therapy Requires a professional	• Removes heavy metals
Toxin-binding agents Can be done at home	• These "vacuum-clean" all kinds of toxins from the body and can help ameliorate symptoms of fatigue, brain fog, pain, and others associated with toxicity.

GINNY'S Story

About fifteen years ago, I started to have weakness in my left leg. I was working as a registered nurse at the time, and I often found myself falling into walls. I also felt unbalanced whenever I walked. A neurologist said that I had peripheral neuropathy and wanted me to take medicine for the symptoms. She told me that fifty percent of the time, doctors don't know what causes neuropathy, but her only solution was to give me medication to manage the symptoms.

Taking medication didn't feel right to me, but I did it anyway, and in the meantime, I discovered Dr. Connealy and the Cancer Center for Healing. Dr. Connealy suspected that I had heavy metal poisoning, and sure enough, the results showed that I had a lot of mercury, cadmium, and other metals in my body. So, she put me on a detoxification program and took IV heavy metal detox treatments, followed by a liter of IV vitamin C. During the IVs, I would also do an ionic foot detox bath.

After about three months of detox therapy, I stopped feeling the tingling in my leg and was no longer falling into walls, and the peripheral neuropathy completely went away.

Then, in 2010, I developed kidney cancer and Dr. Connealy has since been helping me recover from that. I had the kidney with the cancer removed, and conventional tests showed that there was no more cancer, but Dr. Connealy wanted me to do a circulating tumor (CTC) test just to be sure. So I did, and sure enough, there were some CTCs. Whatever cancer cells were left over from the kidney cancer hadn't yet had a chance to get reestablished somewhere else in the body and create a new tumor.

Since the discovery of the CTCs, I've been on several anticancer protocols. My CTC count last September was at 16; now it is at 2, which is very low.

I continue to do detoxification treatments, such as sauna therapy, as part of my morning and evening routine, and I take supplements to keep my immune system functioning and my body alkaline.

CHAPTER 6

Harness the Power of Supplements

IN THIS CHAPTER, YOU WILL LEARN . . .

- Why you should consider nutritional supplements with anticancer properties
- Which supplements support the body and may help eliminate circulating tumor cells (CTCs) and circulating stem cells (CSCs)
- Four foundational supplements that can aid in your cancer fight
- How to identify what supplements your body needs
- The anticancer components of fifteen nutrients

Nutritional and cancer-fighting supplements are an integral part of any comprehensive cancer treatment plan, but, despite claims of miracle cures on the Internet, no supplement alone eliminates cancer. Yet supplements play a very important role in cancer treatment because cancer is continually trying to outsmart whatever you are doing, and supplements can help you attack it from multiple angles. To do this, I would suggest using a variety of targeted supplements, which you and your doctor will want to rotate on a regular basis.

Supplements serve a fourfold purpose in cancer treatment: to detoxify your body, provide it with foundational nutrients, to balance and augment your immune system function, and target circulating tumor cells and/or stem cells. You'll want your doctor to use the lab tests that are described later in this section to determine exactly what supplements you need. If you have cancer, in addition to the few core supplements I recommend for everyone, you'll want to find out what supplements may aid in eliminating the circulating tumor cells (CTCs) and circulating stem cells (CSCs), because chemotherapy and radiation can't kill them, and if you'll recall from Chapter 1, they are responsible for over 95 percent of all metastases.

It is beyond the scope of this book to describe all of the nutrients and supplements that you may need to get well or remain well, so in this chapter, I will primarily be sharing with you the kinds of supplements that help prevent cancer, modulate the immune system, and which have cancer-killing effects upon CSCs, CTCs, and tumor cells. I'll also discuss some core anticancer supplements that we recommend to every single one of our patients and which should form the foundation of any anticancer regimen. These can help strengthen and revitalize the body, but they also possess properties linked with cancer prevention.

Integrative doctors recommend that these nutrients be a part of patients' nutritional regimen, just like eating your spinach and salmon. Even if you choose the conventional route of treatment and do chemotherapy or radiation, you'll still need to take supplements to support and heal your body.

There are literally hundreds of supplements with anticancer properties, but not all of them will work for your particular type of cancer or situation, so you and your doctor will want to do testing to find out which ones you need. Testing is also important because certain supplements are synergistic in their effects; that is, they are more powerful when combined with other types of supplements. So, don't just take random amounts of different supplements, because the ones you think you need may not be the ones that will help you, and they may in fact harm you. RGCC testing is a good way to find out exactly what natural anticancer agents your CTCs and CSCs will respond to.

Finally, it's a good idea to consult with your doctor before taking any of the supplements recommended in this chapter, to make sure that they aren't contraindicated for your particular situation and don't interact with other medications or supplements that you may be taking.

Getting Your Nutrient Levels Tested

Most people with cancer have nutritional deficiencies, so in addition to RGCC testing (which tells you what specific agents your cancer will respond to), you'll also want to do testing to determine what nutrients your body needs to rebuild and repair itself. SpectraCell Laboratories is one great lab used for nutritional testing that your doctor could employ to create a foundational nutritional protocol for you. SpectraCell measures the function of thirty-five nutritional components in your body, including vitamins, antioxidants, minerals, and amino acids. You can have your blood drawn at your local lab, and then mailed out to the SpectraCell lab for analysis and interpretation.

NutrEval by Genova Diagnostics is another lab test that assesses your nutritional status, and like the SpectraCell, it can be done at your local lab. In addition, NutrEval evaluates your gastrointestinal and detoxification functions. Testing to find out what nutrients your body needs is so important because no two people have the same nutritional requirements, and neither do they respond well to the same brands or types of products.

You can do the SpectraCell and many of the other types of tests that we discuss in *The Cancer Revolution* on your own, but like other aspects of treatment, it's best to work with a knowledgeable integrative doctor who can interpret their results and customize a supplement plan for you.

The Four Core Anticancer Supplements

The following four supplements should form the basis of any cancer prevention or treatment plan, along with any other supplements indicated by RGCC, nutritional, and other types of lab testing. You'll want to rely on test results and your doctor's recommendations for the other anticancer supplements described later in this chapter to determine whether those supplements are right for you, and if so, in what amounts.

Vitamin C

Vitamin C may be one of the most powerful immunity-boosting anticancer supplements in nature. As I mentioned in Chapter 3, oral vitamin C has different effects upon the body than does high-dose, intravenous (IV) vitamin C. At lower dosages, vitamin C can help boost immune function. Research suggests vitamin C in high doses may be linked to cancer eradication, as the nutrient can produce lethal hydrogen peroxide inside of tumors, which causes them to self-destruct.[1]

Oral vitamin C is a fantastic supplement that I highly recommend to everyone, for both cancer prevention and treatment, because of its potent immunity-enhancing properties. The late Linus Pauling, who was one of the most influential biochemists in history and a two-time Nobel Prize winner, was among the first scientists to conduct research that suggests high doses of vitamin C may be lethal to cancer. In his book *Vitamin C and Cancer*, he shares detailed accounts of cancer patients who experienced significant increases in their life expectancy, including some complete remissions, as a result of high-dose vitamin C treatments.[2]

The US Recommended Daily Allowance (RDA) for vitamin C is 60 mg daily, with an upper limit of 2000 mg.[3] The RDA guidelines are based on the minimum amount that's needed to prevent scurvy and are not what the body needs to function optimally. The average amount that I recommend to my patients is about 8,000 mg. If you just want to prevent cancer, I recommend taking 4,000 mg daily.

One type of vitamin C you may want to try is liposomal vitamin C, which is encased in phospholipids, or fats that come from sunflower lecithin. The phospholipids increase your body's ability to absorb and utilize the vitamin. Liposomal vitamin C is more expensive than other types of vitamin C, but because it is more bioavailable, your body absorbs and utilizes more of it, so you don't need to take as much. See the Resources section for a list of vitamin C products you can use to get your daily dose.

You'll want to avoid the many vitamin C products that are made from GMO corn, are not necessarily bioavailable to the body, and/or cause gastric distress because they contain no buffers, such as calcium or magnesium. As with all of the other supplements listed in this chapter, you will want to ask your doctor before adjusting your vitamin C intake to make sure that it doesn't interfere with any other supplements or medications that you may be taking.

Vitamin D$_3$

Vitamin D$_3$, which is the most bioavailable form of vitamin D, is one of the most powerful anticancer nutrients in nature. It positively influences over two hundred genes in the body,[4] and can help reduce inflammation, inhibit cancer cells' growth and replication cycle, inhibit new tumor blood vessel growth, and may even induce cancer cell self-destruction. It also may promote the growth of healthy cells.

Nearly all of us could benefit from taking a vitamin D$_3$ supplement. In my experience, anywhere from 5,000 to 15,000 IUs daily can be beneficial, depending on the patient's test results. It's usually safe to take a low dose of vitamin D without getting tested, but it's ideal to have your doctor test you to find out what your current vitamin D levels are so you know exactly how much you need. You want your results to be in the top half of the testing results range, or at 50 to 70 ng/ml. If they are less than that, then this means you need supplemental vitamin D_3. Vitamin D is a very powerful nutrient that acts more like a hormone rather than a vitamin in the body. There may be a few rare situations for which its use is contraindicated. When in doubt, check with your doctor before taking it. See the Resources section for vitamin D product recommendations.

Parent Essential Oils (PEOs)

The third type of supplement you'll want to add to your core regimen is essential fatty acids (EFAs) from parent essential oils (PEOs). PEOs are omega-6 and omega-3 essential fatty acids from linoleic and alpha-linoleic acids. Researcher and PEO developer Brian Peskin, who coined the term "parent essential oils," believes PEOs are the only whole, unadulterated, fully functional forms of the only two essential fats that your body demands.[5] PEOs may help oxygenate the cells and affect the state of cell membranes. When your cell membranes are strong and healthy, your cells become more efficient at uptaking nutrients and expelling waste. They are able to receive more oxygen, which helps your normal cells remain healthy, while encouraging the destruction of the cancerous ones. An insufficient amount of PEOs in your diet can reduce the amount of oxygen in your cells and increase your risk of cancer, so you'll want to make sure to get your EFAs from PEOs.

We recommend that our patients take omega-3 EFAs from supplemental alpha-linoleic acid and omega-6 EFAs from linoleic acid, which come from such foods as walnuts, hazelnuts, sesame seeds, and apricot oil. These can also be purchased in supplement form. In the Resources section I provide some EFA supplement recommendations. EFAs generally produce no side effects.

Pancreatic Proteolytic Enzymes

Pancreatic enzymes can benefit everyone. First, many people have what's called pancreatic insufficiency, which means that their body can't produce sufficient amounts of pancreatic enzymes due to stress, toxins, a bad diet, and other factors. You can find out whether your body is producing sufficient enzymes by doing a couple of simple blood and/or stool tests. The blood tests your doctor will want to order for you are called amylase and lipase, which are two types of enzymes produced by the pancreas and that help show how well your body is producing digestive enzymes. Your doctor may also want to order a stool test that measures elastase, which is an enzyme that digests protein and is another useful measure of pancreatic function.

If you find out that you have pancreatic insufficiency, supplemental enzyme products can help your pancreas digest food and keep it from becoming overtaxed by a poor diet that may be too heavy in protein.

Second, and perhaps more important, pancreatic enzymes may be useful for stripping cancer cells of fibrin, which is an outer coating that shields them from the immune system. When taken on an empty stomach, enzymes like trypsin and chymotrypsin—which are found in some pancreatic enzyme products—help break up this fibrin so your immune system can potentially better detect then help eradicate the cancer.

The suggested benefits of pancreatic enzyme therapy in cancer treatment were first recognized in the early 1900s. A Scottish embryologist named John Beard proposed that pancreatic proteolytic enzymes were the body's main defense against cancer and that taking supplemental enzymes could kill cancer cells. His theory and research on enzyme therapy are published in a monograph entitled *The Enzyme Therapy of Cancer*.[6] Dr. Beard witnessed many thousands of his patients and clients heal from late-stage cancers as a result of taking pancreatic enzymes.

Ultimately, Dr. Beard's findings suggest pancreatic enzymes may be a very powerful supplement, useful for both cancer prevention and cancer treatment, but the amount you would want to take depends on whether you are trying to prevent cancer or beat it, and not all pancreatic enzyme products are created equal. Look for broad-spectrum proteolytic enzyme formulations that contain such enzymes as pancreatin, bromelain, papain, lipase, amylase, trypsin, and alpha-chymotrypsin. In the Resources section I share some suggested enzyme products, along with dosing recommendations. Pancreatic enzyme dosing is an art, so it's best to consult with your integrative doctor to determine what products and amounts are best for your particular situation. Pancreatic enzymes are very safe and generally not contraindicated in most situations, if taken according to product or your doctor's guidelines.

Supplements to Improve Digestion

Many cancer patients may have trouble digesting their food, so it's sometimes recommended that they take hydrochloric acid, digestive enzymes (which can be different than pancreatic proteolytic enzymes), probiotics, and foods containing probiotics, to assist with this process. Whether you are looking to heal from cancer or simply prevent it, you may want to add these to your regimen as well.

Hydrochloric acid helps your stomach break down food, while digestive enzymes in your small intestines further break it down, digest, and assimilate it into your body. Probiotics populate your large and small intestines with beneficial bacteria that may get stripped away as a result of antibiotics in the food supply, pathogenic infections, toxins from the environment, and other factors. A large part of your immune system is found in your gut, so having a healthy gut is crucial. In fact, your intestines contain more immune cells than does any other part of your body! This is little appreciated by people who think the gut's only role is digestion. The intestines and the beneficial organisms that live in them don't just help us digest food; they have many other functions. For instance, they prevent microbes and pathogenic bacteria from invading our body, and help them create essential nutrients and vitamins.

Unfortunately, the health of our guts is often compromised due to environmental toxins, antibiotics, a poor diet, stress, and other factors. This effect may cause a disruption in the "cross talk" between the microbes in the gut and the other cells involved in immune system and metabolic processes.[7]

You can help maintain your gut health by taking a hydrochloric acid supplement, along with digestive enzymes and probiotics, all of which you can purchase at your local health food store. You'll also want to include more fermented foods in your diet because these contain live cultures that can help repopulate your gut with beneficial bacteria and restore a healthy microbial environment there. Use food-based sources of nutrients whenever possible because nutrients from nature are always better than those found in a pill. You will know a product is made from food and not chemicals because the ingredient label will read "food based," "whole food cultured," or something similar. Excellent fermented foods include kefir, sauerkraut, kombucha, and kimchi. See the Resources section for information about where to find a great selection of healthy, delicious fermented food products and probiotic supplements.

Other Anticancer Supplements

Now that you know which supplements are essential for you to take—whether you want to prevent cancer or better fight it—following I share some of the most important patient-specific cancer fighting supplements. These can be powerful and effective immunity-enhancing and cancer-killing supplements that are prescribed based on patients' bioenergetic test results (bioenergetic testing is described in Chapter 2), RGCC, and/or other lab results. You and your doctor should include them in your cancer treatment regimen only if your lab and other test results indicate that you need them. Some of these supplements are also useful for cancer prevention and for health maintenance, but again, it's best to have your doctor first test you to determine whether they would benefit you.

While all of the following supplements are generally very safe to take and contraindicated only in a few situations, all supplements and medications can interact with other supplements and medications, and either potentiate or decrease their effects. In some cases, they can also cause harm to the body, so I strongly encourage you to consult with your doctor before taking them, to learn whether such an interaction may occur for you.

CoQ10

Cancer results from oxidative damage to cells, which is caused by free radicals, or unstable molecules that damage cells. Many of us have huge amounts of free radicals in our bodies, due to environmental toxins, a poor diet, and inflammation. CoQ10 is a potent intracellular antioxidant that quenches free radicals. It also may enhance the activity of macrophages, one of your body's key immune cells that "gobbles up" and digests cellular debris, foreign substances, microbes, and cancer cells in a process called phagocytosis. CoQ10 increases the proliferation of granulocytes, another type of important immune cell.

CoQ10 is generally safe for most people to take. Some researchers are concerned that it might lower the effectiveness of some chemotherapy drugs, so you'll want to consult with your doctor if you are on a chemotherapy regimen. It may also be contraindicated in a few other situations or conditions. See the Resources section for CoQ10 product and dosage recommendations.

Quercetin

Quercetin is a potent antioxidant and immune system modulator famous for its ability to modulate a gene signal called NF-kappaB, which is crucial for helping your body manage stress and inflammation. It has also been shown in many studies to encourage cancer cell self-destruction, inhibit tumor growth, and reduce cancer's resistance to chemotherapy. Studies suggest that quercetin may impact several types of cancer, including esophageal, colorectal, hepatocellular (liver) carcinoma, ovarian, pancreatic, and prostate cancers.[8]

Quercetin also may help chelate, or remove, "transition" heavy metals from the body. These are heavy metals that may have just entered the body but have not yet found a home deep within the tissues.

One highly recommended quercetin product is called Bio-FCTS, from Biotics Research. This product, which is made from buckwheat, also contains other anticancer substances, such as green tea extract, bioflavonoids, and thymus and spleen extracts, all of which boost the immune system. See the Resources section for information about where to obtain this and other quercetin products. Typical dosages of oral quercetin have been found to be safe, but there have been a few reports of kidney damage when it is given via IV, although such reports are rare. Talk to your doctor about possible contraindications and side effects.

Melatonin

Melatonin is yet another powerful antioxidant that is naturally secreted by the pineal gland in your brain at night while you sleep. Many of us don't produce enough melatonin, potentially due to the prevalence of electromagnetic fields (EMFs) in our environment and excessive artificial light exposure at night, among other reasons. Taking supplemental melatonin can help you sleep better, but it is also a powerful anticancer agent.

Research suggests melatonin may have cytotoxic effects upon different types of cancer, including some liver, breast, prostate, lung, and brain cancers. The result of a combined analysis of ten studies on melatonin published in the *Journal of Pineal Research* showed that, in these cases, melatonin lowered the risk of many cancers by up to 34 percent. The lead researcher concluded, "The substantial reduction in risk of death, low adverse events reported and low costs related to this intervention suggest great potential for melatonin in treating cancer."[9]

I'd recommend dosages of 3 to 20 mg of melatonin, depending on the patient's needs. Lower amounts, such as 1 to 3 mg, are usually sufficient for improved sleep, while higher doses—anywhere from 10 to 20 mg—are needed to treat cancer. If you just want to help prevent cancer or get better rest at night, taking 1 to 3 mg is usually sufficient. To find whether it's an appropriate treatment for your particular type of cancer, you'll want your doctor to order an RGCC test. If so, he or she can then determine how much you need for that purpose. See the Resources section for product recommendations and further information about dosing guidelines.

Melatonin is usually safe when it is taken according to established guidelines, and it is a very beneficial supplement for most people. It may be occasionally contraindicated in a few situations. Talk to your doctor before adding it to your regimen.

Artemisinin

Artemisinin is derived from an herb called artemisia, or wormwood. It has been widely studied, especially in recent years, for its suggested anticancer effects. Research suggests it may help disable cancer cells by reacting with the iron inside them that helps them grow, and by triggering free radical production. The free radicals aid in destroying the cancer cell membrane and, with that, the cancer cell. Artemisinin also oxygenates the body.

Studies suggest artemisinin could have anticancer effects upon fifty-five different types of cancer cells, ranging from leukemia, to colon, lung, and breast cancer cells, and fibrosarcomas (cancers derived from fibrous connective tissue). It has also been proven to kill cancers that have traditionally been resistant to chemotherapy.[10] See the Resources section for product recommendations and typical dosages. Artemisinin is a safe supplement, but, as with all of the supplements in this section, it should be taken only if your doctor and test results indicate that you need it. The side effects and contraindications of artemisinin are generally few. If you have a history of liver disease, you should absolutely consult with your doctor before using it, as there have been a few reports of liver problems among those who have used artemisinin, especially at higher dosages.

Garlic

Garlic is a delicious food linked with a reduced risk of cancer. It is also a powerful medicinal supplement. According to the National Cancer Institute, studies suggest that consuming garlic may reduce the risk of developing many kinds of cancers, especially gastrointestinal cancers, such as stomach and colon cancers, but also esophageal, pancreatic, and breast cancers.[11]

Like all of the other supplements described in this chapter, garlic may be toxic to cancer cells, but is a great addition to any anticancer protocol because it also strengthens the immune system. People who eat garlic tend to have increased natural killer (NK) cell counts, which is one of the body's front-line immune cells involved in fighting cancer. Garlic is also thought to help your liver detoxify and potentially remove cancer-causing compounds, as well as stimulate the production of glutathione, one of your body's most important antioxidants. A meta-analysis of combined studies on the effects of garlic on gastric cancers, published in January 2015, revealed that consuming *any* amount of garlic helped prevent all kinds of gastric cancers, although the more you take, the greater the effects.[12]

So, enjoy lots of garlic in your food, and if testing indicates, use higher amounts in supplement form as part of your anticancer treatment regimen. Garlic is a wonderful food and when taken in supplement form, is also safe when taken according to product guidelines. Because garlic lowers blood pressure, higher doses may be contraindicated in people with low blood pressure. See your doctor to discuss potential side effects and contraindications.

Green Tea Extract

Green tea contains chemicals called polyphenols, which have potent anticancer properties. The most famous of these is called EGCG, a powerful free radical scavenger and anti-inflammatory agent that could protect cells from DNA damage that eventually may lead to cancer. But it also may directly induce apoptosis, or cancer cell self-destruction, and stop tumor blood vessel development. EGCG's antioxidant effects are considered by some researchers to be more powerful than those of either vitamin E or C.

EGCG rarely causes side effects, although there have been occasional reports of indigestion and nausea with it, and rarely, liver problems, especially when it is given in higher doses. Again, talk to your doctor for more information on the side effects and contraindications of EGCG that may impact you individually.

You can purchase green tea extract over the counter. See the Resources section for product recommendations.

Indole-3-Carbinol

Indole-3-carbinol (I3C) is a chemical found in cruciferous vegetables, such as cauliflower, cabbage, broccoli, Brussels sprouts, cauliflower, and kale. It partially blocks the effects of chemicals that have xenoestrogenic effects upon the body and which can increase your risk for some types of cancers, especially reproductive cancers such as those of the breast, uterus, cervix, and prostate.

You can do hormone testing to determine whether excess estrogen or xenoestrogens are playing a role in your disease or putting you at a greater risk of contracting certain types of cancer. The Estronex Profile is one test that can do this by measuring how well your body metabolizes and eliminates estrogens. If you find that you have too many "bad estrogens" in your body, you can help reduce their impact by increasing your intake of vegetables that contain I3C, or by taking an over-the-counter I3C supplement, which you can get at your local health food store. I3C is a very safe supplement that causes no side effects. If you take any medications that are broken down in the liver, indole-3-carbinol may increase their breakdown rate and decrease their effectiveness, so consult your doctor before taking it if you also take medications.

Curcumin

In Chapter 3, I mentioned that curcumin is a powerful anti-inflammatory chemical that comes from the popular Asian spice turmeric, which has a number of anticancer properties. Refer to Chapter 3 for more information about its potential role in cancer treatment.

Many integrative doctors do IV curcumin treatments or, in some cases, recommend oral curcumin. Most people can safely take high amounts of oral curcumin for cancer prevention, but if you or your doctor wish to incorporate it into your treatment plan, it's best to get tested to find out what dosage would be best for you.

Curcumin isn't contraindicated in most health conditions or situations and can be safely taken with most other supplements and medications. Rarely, allergic reactions may occur. If you are allergic to plants in the ginger family, or yellow food coloring, which often contains curcumin, consult your doctor before taking it.

Essiac Tea

In 1922, a nurse named Rene Caisse, from Ontario, Canada, learned that one of her patients had recovered from breast cancer by taking an Indian herbal tea from an Ojibwa medicine man. She apparently then used the recipe to treat her aunt's stomach cancer and found it to be so successful that she opened a clinic and treated thousands of patients with injections and tea preparations created from the herbs. She named the combination of the herbs Essiac, which is her last name spelled backward.

Essiac is most commonly taken as a tea or in capsules and consists of four main herbs: burdock root, slippery elm inner bark, sheep sorrel, and Indian rhubarb root, all of which have cytotoxic, or cancer-killing properties.

Essiac also improves immune system function, relieves pain, restores energy, detoxifies the body, increases appetite, reduces inflammation, and eliminates excess mucus in the organs—among other things.

Some media have reported that Essiac tea is a controversial treatment, but in my personal experience I have seen that it can be a powerful tool to help prevent cancer, and some patients' RGCC tests have produced results that suggest that's the case.

You can purchase Essiac as a tea or in supplement form, for both cancer prevention and treatment purposes. However, not all brands of Essiac products are created equal, and some may be downright ineffective, so if you decide to try Essiac, purchase the tea or capsules through a reputable company, such as EssiacProducts.com, which uses the original formula created by Rene Caisse in their products. See the Resources section for information on where to purchase Essiac tea/supplements and for dosing guidelines.

Essiac tea and supplements are generally safe when taken according to product guidelines. They may be contraindicated in a few health conditions, such as kidney disease and colitis, or if you have a bowel obstruction or diarrhea. You may also want to consult with your doctor before taking Essiac if you are diabetic or on blood-thinning medication. Talk to your doctor before taking Essiac tea.

Medicinal Mushrooms

Medicinal mushrooms are used worldwide to treat cancer and enhance immune system function. Shiitake, maitake, ganoderma, reishi, and cordyceps are a few of the most widely used mushrooms. They have been used for millennia in parts of Asia, and we also use them as part of some of our patients' anticancer regimens. Mushrooms have immunity-modulating, anti-cancer, antiviral, anti-inflammatory, and liver protective properties.

It is beyond the scope of this book to describe the anticancer benefits of all the different types of mushrooms, but one recommended combination mushroom product is called Host Defense My Community Capsules. This product contains seventeen powerful mushroom species that have anticancer effects and promote immune system health. It is a great addition to any anticancer protocol or cancer prevention regimen. Other well-researched and quality mushroom products include those created by Tsu-Tsair Chi, a PhD biochemist and doctor whose formulas are used by many thousands of doctors worldwide. For more information on these and other recommended mushroom products, see the Resources section. Because there are such a wide variety of mushrooms on the market, each with its own unique anticancer benefits, it's best to consult with your doctor and test to determine which of these might be best for your unique situation, and in what dosages.

Other Cytotoxic Nutrients

Other natural substances that may be effective for treating many cancers and that studies suggest have anticancer benefits, include:

- Aloe vera
- Amygdalin
- Cat's claw
- Low-dose naltrexone
- Lycopene
- Mistletoe
- Modified citrus pectin
- Poly MVA
- Rerio (Guna)
- Resveratrol
- Salicinium
- Salvesterol
- Thymex
- Tocotrienols and vitamin E
- Vascu-Statin

Ask your doctor to order an RGCC test, or do a bioenergetic test (see Chapter 2) to find out whether some or any of these would be beneficial for treating the particular type of cancer that you have.

SUPPLEMENTS		
Core Supplements (Everyone)	**Benefits**	**Recommended Dosage**
Vitamin C	• At lower dosages, boosts immune function and lowers inflammation • At higher doses and when given by IV, kills cancer cells	Per your doctor's recommendations (See Resources for more detailed product and dosage information.)

SUPPLEMENTS continued

Core Supplements (Everyone)	Benefits	Recommended Dosage
Vitamin D	• Positively influences more than 200 genes • Reduces inflammation • Inhibits cancer cell growth and its replication cycle • Inhibits the formation of tumor blood vessels • Induces cancer cell self-destruction	Per your doctor's recommendations (See Resources for more detailed product and dosage information.)
Parent essential oils (PEOs)	• Oxygenates the cells • Helps heal healthy cells and cell membranes	Per your doctor's or the package recommendations (See Resources for more detailed product and dosage information.)
Proteolytic pancreatic enzymes	• Strips cancer cells of fibrin so that they become more vulnerable to attack by treatments	Per your doctor's recommendations (See Resources for more detailed product and dosage information.)

Supplements for Digestion

Hydrochloric acid and digestive enzymes	• Breaks down, digests, and assimilates food	Take according to the product instructions.
Probiotic food and supplements	• Populates the large and small intestines with beneficial bacteria, which play a powerful role in immune function	Take according to the product instructions.

Anticancer Supplements (Take only if recommended by your doctor.)

CoQ10	• Quenches free radicals • Enhances the activity of macrophages, a key immune cell that "gobbles up" cancer cells • Increases the proliferation of granulocytes, another immune cell involved in fighting cancer	Take 300–400 mg daily.
Quercetin	• Quenches free radicals • Lowers inflammation • Encourages cancer cell self-destruction • Inhibits tumor growth • Reduces cancer's resistance to chemotherapy	Take according to your doctor's or the package instructions.
Melatonin	• Lowers the risk for many types of cancer, by up to 34% • Has a variety of potent anticancer properties	Take 1–3 mg before bedtime to improve sleep. For cancer treatment, take 10–20 mg before bedtime, or according to your doctor's instructions.

continues

SUPPLEMENTS continued		
Core Supplements (Everyone)	Benefits	Recommended Dosage
Artemisinin	• Disables cancer cells by reacting with the iron inside them that helps them grow, and by producing cancer-destroying free radicals • Oxygenates the body • Effective for treating 55 types of cancer cells • Kills cancers that are resistant to chemotherapy	Take 2 capsules 2x daily.
Garlic	• Improves natural killer (NK) cell function, one of the body's front-line immune cells involved in fighting cancer. • Helps the liver detoxify and remove cancer-causing compounds • Stimulates the production of glutathione, one of the body's most important antioxidants • Helps prevent all kinds of gastric cancers	
Green tea extract	• Quenches free radicals. Its antioxidant effects may be more powerful than those of vitamins E and C • Protects cells from DNA damage • Kills cancer cells and stops tumor blood vessel production, which tumors use to get their food	Take as directed on the product label, or 2 capsules, 2x/day.
Indole-3-carbinol (I3C)	• Partially blocks the effects of chemicals that encourage the growth of reproductive cancers such as breast, uterine, cervical, and prostate	Take 1 capsule, 2x/day.
Curcumin	• Counteracts the initial processes in the body that lead to cancer, as well as the mechanisms that allow tumors to grow • Interferes with the development of cancer stem cells • Enhances the effectiveness of some types of chemotherapy • Disrupts the production of inflammatory chemicals that initiate cancer development • Is as effective as some pharmaceutical drugs for treating cancers of the prostate, colon, breast, liver, esophagus, and mouth	Take 500 mg, 3x day.

continues

SUPPLEMENTS	continued	
Essiac tea	• Kills cancer cells • Improves immune system function • Relieves pain • Restores energy • Detoxifies the body • Increases appetite • Reduces inflammation • Eliminates excess mucus in the organs	Take as directed on the product label.
Medicinal mushrooms	• Have immune modulating and anti-inflammatory properties • Kill cancer cells • Protect the liver	Take as directed on the product label.
Other cytotoxic nutrients	See page 108.	Take as directed on the product label.

MEG'S Story

I was diagnosed with stage 2B breast cancer in 2001. I chose to do chemotherapy, radiation, and surgery. After that, I tested negative for cancer for eleven years, and all of my labs were normal until October 2012, when I was diagnosed with a stage 4 breast cancer that had spread to my liver. I did a half-dose, four-month chemotherapy regimen starting in November 2012. Since I hadn't tolerated the chemotherapy well the first time around, my doctor cut the dosage in half. In the meantime, I went to see Dr. Connealy.

Dr. Connealy encouraged me to continue chemotherapy and gave me some anticancer and immunity-supportive supplements to take at the same time. She did limbic stress assessment (LSA) testing and lab testing to determine which supplements and products would work best for me. We used, and are still using, everything possible to beat the cancer.

I take turmeric supplements, pancreatic enzymes, quercetin, and plant-based parent essential oils (PEOs), to name a few. I drink ginger and turmeric lemonade daily. I include and rotate nearly all of the supplements that have anticancer, anti-inflammatory, and immunity-building properties. Since the cancer was in my liver and has affected how well it functions, I use an herbal combination to help regulate my blood sugar.

Dr. Connealy had also noticed that one of my lab numbers was high, due to a parasite infection, so she referred me to a herbologist who gave me herbal tinctures to get rid of it. He mentioned that he'd never seen a breast cancer patient without parasites. Turns out, they were in my liver, so I've been using a tincture for several months and seem to be making progress. I notice that I am feeling more energy and less pain in my liver.

I've been on Dr. Connealy's regimen since October 2012, and most of my cancer markers and lab results, including my CTCs and CSCs, and naga-lase, have greatly improved. My liver used to be covered in lesions; now they are gone and everything is functioning well.

Taking supplements has been essential to my recovery, along with detoxifying my body. I do dry body brushing, laser light therapy, yoga, and fasting, among other things. I eat according to my metabolic type and pre-pare foods according to the wisdom of Weston A. Price. I exercise regularly and develop emotional/spiritual/mental strength and stability. Stress plays a bigger role in disease than one might think. We all need to slow down. Life is precious, and we can choose to enjoy every day. That is what will ultimately change our health.

CHAPTER 7

Get Moving to Get Well

IN THIS CHAPTER, YOU WILL LEARN . . .

- How exercise reduces your cancer risk and can help combat cancer
- The top ten anticancer benefits of exercise
- How to find an exercise or daily activity for your fitness level

When you have cancer, the last thing that you may feel like doing is exercising. Everyone knows exercise promotes health, but you may not be motivated to do it because you don't feel great, are busy, or simply don't know that it can impact your recovery just as much as any treatment, nutrient, or detoxification program.

Yet exercise plays an extremely important role in cancer prevention and in battling cancer. Exercise isn't just good for you; it is medicine for your body.

Surprisingly, most oncologists don't encourage their patients to exercise, but according to the National Cancer Institute (NCI), exercise is safe and beneficial for most people with cancer to do while they are undergoing treatment. Also, engaging in physical activity after a cancer diagnosis is associated with a longer life span and a reduced risk of cancer recurrence among people who have many types of cancer, including breast, colorectal, prostate, lung, and ovarian cancers.[1]

Studies on people with breast and colon cancer show that those who exercise regularly have *half* the recurrence, or relapse rate of those who don't exercise.[2] So, once you are in remission, exercise can serve to help keep you there. While these studies didn't include other types of cancer, hundreds of other studies, most of which can be accessed on medical research databases, such as PubMed.org, have shown that moderate exercise has similar benefits for other types of cancer.

Exercise also reduces cancer risk. More than fifty studies on the relationship between colon cancer and physical activity consistently suggest that adults who increase either the intensity, duration, or frequency of their daily physical activity reduce their risk of developing colon cancer by 30 to 40 percent, compared to those who are sedentary.[3] And over sixty studies published worldwide demonstrate that women who are physically active have a lowered risk of developing breast cancer than do sedentary women, but the degree of risk reduction varies widely, between 20 and 80 percent, depending on a variety of factors.[4] While many of these studies suggest that you need to exercise for thirty to sixty minutes daily at a moderate- to high-intensity level,[5] one study found that women who exercised moderately (the equivalent of walking for three to five hours per week at an average pace) after a diagnosis of breast cancer still had improved survival rates compared with more sedentary women. The benefit was particularly pronounced in women with hormone-responsive tumors.[6]

Other studies on the correlation between exercise and other types of cancer have produced similar results. So, even if you can't go to the gym, if you are just able to get out and walk daily for twenty to thirty minutes you'll decrease your risk of getting cancer, or increase your chances of recovering from it.

Finally, exercise has also been shown to reduce the side effects of some chemotherapy drugs, so if you are doing chemotherapy treatments, exercise can help you feel better after treatments. One study on mice that had received a chemo drug called doxorubicin, which negatively affects the heart, showed that when the mice were subjected to physical exercise, the mitochondria of their heart functioned better because the exercise prevented the drug from causing them oxidative stress and damage. That study's findings should be taken with a grain of salt as the research involved mice, which are different from humans, but ultimately this conclusion suggests exercise may help protect your body against the toxic effects of some drugs.[7]

The Top Ten Anticancer Benefits of Exercise

Exercise provides numerous benefits to your body that may be powerful for reducing cancer risk, improving health outcomes, and reducing cancer recurrences. After you read about these benefits, you just may find yourself further motivated to get up and get moving!

1. Exercise powerfully boosts immune function. One of the most important benefits of exercise is that it enhances your body's immune function. It does this by improving the circulation of immune cells throughout the body, so that they can more easily get to their destination, which are the cancer cells. The better that your immune cells circulate throughout your body, the more efficient they may be at locating and attacking the cancer cells, as well as other immunity-suppressing agents, such as bacteria and viruses.

Research also suggests exercise may help improve immune function by stimulating the activity of some types of cancer-killing immune cells; particularly, natural killer (NK), monocytes, and granulocytes.[8] Natural killer cells identify and eliminate tumor cells and are one of your body's frontline defenses against cancer, while monocytes and granulocytes also play a role in destroying cancer cells. For example, monocytes can become macrophages, a type of immune cell that literally swallows cancer cells whole!

2. Exercise stimulates your lymphatic system. The lymphatic system helps immune cells get to where they need to go, and may help shuttle cancer-fighting nutrients into the cells and carry cancer-causing toxins out of them. Rebounding, jump-roping, or bouncing up and down on a large ball are some great exercises that are particularly effective for helping you get your lymph fluid moving. If you are bedbound, you can have someone massage you, and this will accomplish the same thing. Or, if you aren't strong enough or have another physical limitation that keeps you from being able to rebound or jump rope, you can stimulate your lymphatic system with a Chi Machine, which is a device that moves your body from side to side in a fishlike fashion while you lie on the floor. You can purchase a Chi Machine online at various retailers, such as Chi Machine International. See the Resources section for more information. Other types of exercise stimulate the lymphatic system to varying degrees, and almost all types of movement stimulate blood flow throughout the body.

3. Exercise increases oxygen and nutrient delivery to your cells, including your brain. As we've discussed throughout this book, cancer can't thrive in an oxygen-rich environment, so exercise directly causes cancer cell death. It also nourishes and invigorates your healthy cells and helps them eliminate waste. Exercise is a great way to add oxygen therapy to your regimen, especially if you can't afford or don't have access to a hyperbaric chamber or other in-clinic oxygen treatments.

4. Exercise drives down your insulin levels. Insulin is a hormone that controls how our body uses and stores energy from food, but it is also a growth factor that signals cancer cells to divide and multiply rapidly. It may even increase the levels of other growth factors that play a role in cancer development and progression, so having too much insulin circulating around in your bloodstream isn't a good thing.

Many of us nowadays are insulin-resistant due to the Standard American Diet (SAD), environmental toxins, and stress. This means that our cells don't readily respond anymore to the normal actions of insulin, which causes our pancreas to work hard to produce more of it, which then leads to excessive amounts in the bloodstream. The good news is you can help correct insulin resistance with a proper diet and exercise, and many studies prove this. For instance, one twelve-week study on obese women, the results of which were published in 2014 in the *Journal of Exercise Nutrition and Biochemistry*, suggested that when a group of women walked for fifty to seventy minutes three times per week, they lost weight in their abdomen, and their blood glucose test results improved. Abdominal fat and abnormal blood glucose levels are both indicators of insulin resistance, so, based on these findings, reducing abdominal fat and normalizing blood glucose levels with exercise may be powerful for lowering insulin levels.[9]

5. Exercise causes you to sweat and remove toxins. Whenever you engage in any kind of relatively strenuous activity, you will perspire or sweat. Sweating helps remove cancer-linked toxins from your body, just like a sauna, and can be just as powerful for detoxifying your body as a sauna. Until recently, few scientific studies proved that sweating actually cleanses the body of toxins. But a groundbreaking study, published in 2011 in the *Archives of Environmental and Contamination Toxicology*, revealed that many toxic elements are preferentially excreted from the body via sweat. The researchers concluded, "Induced sweating appears to be a potential method for elimination of many toxic elements from the human body."[10] Two additional studies published in 2012 suggested that sweating enhances the elimination of dangerous hormone-disrupting petrochemicals, such as BPA (which are found in plastics) and phthalates, both of which have been linked to breast cancer.[11]

6. Exercise reduces estrogen-producing body fat. In Chapter 2, I mentioned that when you have too many xenoestrogens (toxic chemical compounds that mimic the activity of estrogen) in your body, then this may facilitate the growth of some cancers. An imbalance of any kind of hormone can potentially increase cancer risk or cause some cancers to grow, but we know that having too much estrogen can contribute to the growth of some kinds of cancer, especially reproductive cancers, such as breast, ovarian, cervical, and prostate cancers.

The late Rose E. Frisch, former associate professor of population sciences emerita at the Harvard School of Public Health, did a study in the 1980s comparing the incidence of reproductive cancers in female college athletes with that of nonathletes. She and her fellow researchers surveyed 5,398 women aged 21 to 82.3, and found that in every age group, the nonathletes had more cancers of the reproductive system, such as uterine, ovarian, and cervical cancer, than the athletes. She also found that the nonathletes had approximately twice the risk of developing breast cancer.[12]

Dr. Frisch believed that one of the reasons the athletes had a lower risk and incidence of cancer was that they had less body fat. Fat acts like an endocrine-producing organ because it stores and releases estrogen into the body, so when you lose fat, you also lose one of your body's main sources of potentially harmful estrogens. Body fat also converts some hormones, such as testosterone and DHEA, to estrogen, so because the athletes made less estrogen than the nonathletes, this protected them against some types of cancer.

7. Exercise may thin your blood and reduce red blood cell clumping. When your red blood cells are clumped together and your blood becomes too thick, cancer-killing immune cells, oxygen, and nutrients can't move as easily about the bloodstream and reach their target cells. The results of a meta-analysis of studies from 1950 to 2010 suggested exercise improved the condition of the study participants' blood, including its thickness, and to keep red blood cells from clumping together.[13] In this way, exercise acts as a natural anticoagulant.

8. Exercise reduces stress. Many of us underestimate the impact of stress upon our lives and so ignore it, instead of finding ways to manage it. It can be tempting to do nothing and just hope it will magically go away. Often, after a rough day at work, all I really want to do is escape from the pressures of the day and tune everything out, but I will often exercise instead. I might go for a jog or find some stairs to climb—basically anything that will get my heart rate up, fill my lungs with oxygen, and help me feel good.

You don't have to jog or climb stairs, but you'll want to do something to keep stress from accumulating in your body because stress can be one of the biggest contributing factors to cancer, as you will see in Chapter 8. Exercise is one of the best ways to manage stress because it causes your body to produce mood-enhancing chemicals called endorphins (when the exercise is moderately intense), and to release excess cortisol, which contributes to anxiety and immunity suppression.

In my experience, whenever someone comes to me with a long list of symptoms, such as irritability, fatigue, sleep problems, repeated colds or infections, high blood pressure, memory loss, weight gain, or cravings for carbohydrates and sweets, the first thing that occurs to me is that they probably have high stress and high levels of cortisol. Cortisol is a hormone produced by the adrenal glands during times of high stress. Together with adrenaline, cortisol mobilizes your body for a "fight or flight" situation, at the same time that it suppresses your digestive and immune systems, so it's not something that you want hanging around for weeks or months at a time. But when you live with chronic, unremitting stress for long periods of time, your body endlessly produces high amounts of this hormone, which in turn may increase your risk for many types of illnesses, including cancer.

Now consider this: For every thirty minutes of exercise you do, you will neutralize twelve hours of accumulated stress in your body. So, getting out and about to take a walk, doing some yoga, or cleaning your car will help you to release a full day of pent-up stress.

9. Exercise relieves depression and insomnia. When you get depressed, often the last thing you may want to do is exercise, but it truly is one of the best medicines for depression. As I mentioned, whenever you engage in any moderately intense exercise, your body releases endorphins, which trigger positive feelings. The sensation that often follows a run or workout is often described as a "runner's high," and can be accompanied by a positive and energizing outlook on life.

Even if you can't do moderately intense exercise, other types of exercise will still rev up the production of some of your body's mood- and sleep-enhancing chemicals, such as serotonin, norepinephrine, and dopamine, which are produced primarily in your brain and gut. These chemicals are responsible for regulating your mood, sleep patterns, and energy—among other things. Depression and insomnia have been linked to cancer because they suppress the immune system, so by increasing your body's production of these mood-enhancing and sleep-inducing chemicals, you can help give your immune system a boost.

10. Exercise reduces inflammation and the risk of developing colorectal cancer. Physical activity helps move food through the bowels, so that the harmful chemical byproducts of food and metabolic waste, which cause colorectal cancer, move out of the body more quickly. The less time that metabolic waste remains in your bowels, the less likely you may be to develop a colorectal cancer. Indeed, many studies, including the two that were cited at the beginning of this chapter, have suggested that exercise reduces the risk and recurrences of colorectal cancer.

Your Anticancer Exercise Regimen

You may be cringing because you aren't accustomed to exercise. Maybe you are too weak to go to the gym or engage in strenuous activity. That's okay! The important thing is that you move, and do at least an hour of what I call "nonexercising activity" daily. This can include such things as washing dishes, cleaning your house, or folding laundry because even household tasks require energy and get you moving. If you are stronger, it's ideal to do thirty to sixty minutes of an exercise that you enjoy, three to five times per week (and do less-strenuous activities on the other days), whether that's walking, Qigong, tai chi, yoga, resistance training, biking, weightlifting, exercising with a large stretchy band, swimming, or another activity (for more on additional benefits of Qigong and yoga, see Chapter 8).

The main thing is to just move around for thirty to sixty minutes every day. For example, just getting up from your computer or sofa and taking a series of five-minute breaks throughout the day to go for short walks or do some stretching exercises can be beneficial. Break up your exercise time so you're not sitting around all day. If taking a short walk multiple times a day is too exhausting, just start with a single five-minute walk, because some exercise is better than no exercise. You can gradually add five minutes to that every week until you are up to twenty to thirty minutes of movement daily. Over time, you could build up to doing a short stretching session first thing in the morning, then taking a five- or ten-minute walk after breakfast, lunch, and/or dinner, and finishing the day off with a little yoga or tai chi before bedtime.

The most important thing is simply committing to doing something. And if you miss a day of exercise, don't beat yourself up and conclude that you've failed at this aspect of your wellness regimen. Just get up and start again the next day!

It can also be helpful to change up your routine so that you don't get bored. Rather than going to the gym every day, take a walk one day; get on a mini-trampoline or rebounder another day; clean your house, or do some yoga. Do activities that you enjoy so you are more likely to stick with them.

If you aren't able to move because you are bedridden or in a wheelchair, or have a physical handicap that prevents you from exercising, massage therapy can provide some of the same benefits as exercise because it stimulates the movement of blood, lymph, and immune cells throughout the body, and helps oxygenate the tissues. You can hire a massage therapist, or simply ask a caregiver or family member to give you a twenty-minute massage daily.

FIND AN ACTIVITY FOR YOUR FITNESS LEVEL

If you are bedbound, in a wheelchair, or immobile . . .	If your energy and stamina are limited and you can do mild- to moderate-intensity exercise . . .	If you're able to do moderate- to high-intensity exercise . . .
Get a massage 3–5x/week.	Stretch for 5–10 minutes.	Stretch for 5–10 minutes.
Do some leg lifts or arm raises in bed or move whatever parts of your body that you are able to move (daily).	Do light yoga exercises (take a class or follow a video) for 20–30 minutes, 3x/week.	Take a yoga class for 30–60 minutes, 3–5x/week.
Use a Chi Machine to stimulate your lymphatic system (see www.theChiMachine.com).	Walk for 10–30 minutes, 3–4/ week.	Walk for 30–60 minutes, 4–6x/ week.
	Fold laundry for 30 minutes.	Lift weights for 30–60 minutes.
	Clean house for 30–60 minutes.	Cycle/swim for 30–60 minutes, 3–5x/week.
	Take a Qigong class 2x/week.	Take a Qigong class 3x/week.
	Take a tai chi class 2x/week.	Take a tai chi class 3x/week.
	Rebound on a mini-trampoline for 5–20 minutes.	Rebound on a mini-trampoline for 20–30 minutes.

Exercise for Life

Exercise is a powerful anticancer treatment that can in many cases be just as essential for becoming or remaining cancer-free as any chemotherapeutic regimen, diet, or supplement. Your body was designed to move, not just sit around all day long, so I encourage you to get into the habit of incorporating some movement into your daily routine. I guarantee you'll not only feel better, but you'll also strengthen your body, stimulate your immune system, and protect yourself against cancer in ways that no medication can.

BOB'S Story

About four years ago, I was diagnosed with prostate cancer, but I'm healthy now because I followed Dr. Connealy's treatment regimen and have always been very active. I'm sixty-three years old, and before I used to see Dr. Connealy I would go to a Pilates class three times per week and play golf on the weekends. But when Dr. Connealy told me that diet, exercise, and my attitude were the most important things I needed to address to be well, I became motivated to keep exercising, and I decided to increase my activity level even more. I now go to an exercise class five days a week for an hour and a half each time, and wow, what a difference it makes in how I feel! In fact, I've never felt better in my life.

I like going to exercise classes because they help me be committed and accountable. Also, classes are a social activity, which makes me happy because I get to be around other people and stay fit at the same time. I've found exercise to be good for my mind, too. Most of the people in the classes that I take are half my age, but I am able to keep up with them and I run circles around the fifty- and sixty-year-olds.

Whenever I miss a week of exercise, I always feel a change in my body. I'm not as loose or supple, and things don't feel quite right. So, I'm always glad whenever I can stay on a regimen because then I wake up feeling good, I'm flexible and loose, and my joints aren't tight. And while I can do a lot, I don't try to keep up with an eighteen- or twenty-year-old, because I'm not eighteen or twenty. I just go to the classes to enjoy myself and stay in shape.

Besides exercise, I also meditate daily and quiet my mind, and this helps keep me grounded. Cancer changed my attitude about life. I realize that every day on this planet is special and that life here isn't going to last forever. Before cancer, I used to go through life thinking that nothing would ever change, and that there was never any urgency to do anything, but I now wake up and appreciate and enjoy every single day because we never know how long we will have on this earth.

CHAPTER 8

Reduce Stress and Reclaim Your Life

IN THIS CHAPTER, YOU WILL LEARN . . .

- How stress suppresses your immune system and can contribute to the onset of cancer or exacerbate the disease
- Ten super stress-reduction strategies for every schedule, budget, and fitness level

In small amounts, stress can be invigorating and uplifting, especially when it is related to a happy event or life change, such as buying a home or getting married. But living with long-term, negative stress—such as the uncertainty of a serious illness like cancer, or financial difficulties—can take a toll on your health.

According to the National Cancer Institute (NCI), studies suggest that psychological stress can affect immune function and tumor growth. At least one study has shown that when mice implanted with human tumors were confined or isolated from other mice—conditions that increase stress—their tumors were more likely to grow and metastasize.[1] Stress encourages cancer development because it suppresses your body's production of immune cells. Stress also releases hormones that promote inflammation and cancer growth, such as cortisol and norepinephrine.

Norepinephrine can stimulate tumor cells to produce compounds that break down the tissue around the tumor cells so they can more easily move through the bloodstream, and in turn create new tumors in other parts of the body. Norepinephrine has also been found to stimulate the growth of VEGF, a chemical responsible for tumor blood vessel development. Tumors use these blood vessels to get their food.[2]

Cortisol increases inflammation and suppresses immune cell production and function. Even more astounding, too much cortisol can actually signal your immune cells to stop working! A meta-analysis on the relationship between stress and illness published in the *Malaysian Journal of Medical Sciences* revealed that chronic and acute stress appear to promote tumor growth and suppress natural killer (NK) cell activity.[3] If you'll recall, your natural killer (NK) cells are one of your body's frontline defenses against cancer.

While stress comes from many sources, in my clinical experience I've found stress that comes from emotional conflicts plays a particularly important role in the development of *every single one* of patients' illnesses. Often, these emotional conflicts don't just relate to cancer or a cancer diagnosis, but also to relationship problems, either past or present. Whether it's a bad marriage or an abusive parent-child relationship or a conflict with a sibling, the stressful emotions that are associated with such situations can create internal conflicts that have a tremendous influence upon your health. If you are repressing long-held emotions and/or are carrying significant unresolved conflicts within yourself, stress is brewing in your body.

Not every stressful event will make you sick, but I encourage you to ask yourself, God, a trusted counselor, or someone who knows you well whether there is an emotional conflict that needs to be resolved in your life so it doesn't manifest as physical symptoms. If so, resolving that conflict will be just as important for your recovery or continued wellness as eating your vegetables, taking your anticancer supplements, getting chemotherapy, or having surgery.

Fortunately, our staff at the Center has discovered some powerful, effective solutions for reducing stress and resolving emotional conflicts, and we have observed our patients heal faster from cancer when they do them. A few of these tools require the assistance of a qualified health care practitioner, but most you can do by yourself at home.

They are powerful because they don't work just at the level of your mind but also on your body—because stress isn't stored just in your mind but also in your organs, tissues, and so on. Most of the tools I describe in this chapter can help you find freedom from stress, as well as from the emotions that can accompany it, such as depression, anxiety, anger, and fear.

There is something for everyone in this chapter. No matter your schedule, finances, or fitness level, I believe that you will be able to find a stress-reduction strategy or two here that will help you get through each day with less anxiety and greater peace of mind, and which will help you tremendously in your wellness journey.

Yoga

Yoga is an ancient physical and spiritual discipline that utilizes a combination of postures, rhythmic breathing, and meditation to reduce stress and promote health. When you do yoga, you tend to forget about your worries because you're focusing on multiple things simultaneously: on meditating, breathing, and your posture. Yoga takes you outside of yourself because it requires you to focus and concentrate, which helps your body, mind, and spirit to align. So, the meditation aspect of yoga can help you release challenging emotions by helping you detach from the things of the world, quiet your mind, and focus and connect with God, or the divine.

If you prefer not to meditate, the stretches and strengthening exercises involved in yoga can still be tremendously beneficial for helping you release stress and promote wellness in your body. Among its many physical benefits, yoga increases energy, strength, and flexibility, improves circulation, relieves pain, stimulates immune function, and produces a sense of peace and relaxation, all through the use of movement, breath, and resistance. And, of course, it helps free you from stress and anxiety by quieting your mind, inducing your body's relaxation response, releasing mood-enhancing brain chemicals, and by enabling you to focus your thoughts.

Yoga is increasingly being used as an adjunct cancer therapy in integrative medical clinics worldwide for its stress-releasing, healing, and rehabilitation benefits. So, if your body has been weakened by treatments, yoga can also help you with your rehabilitation process.

Many studies support yoga for healing from cancer and stress reduction. One 2013 study conducted by the University of Calgary suggested that people who practiced yoga had better moods, less stress, and an improved quality of life.[4] Another study revealed yoga may have even more positive effects upon mood than walking.[5] A third study at the University of Texas, MD Anderson Cancer Center, found that cancer patients with lymphoma who did Tibetan yoga slept deeper and longer, and didn't need to use sleep medication as often as those who didn't do it.[6] By now you know that improved sleep translates into lower cortisol levels, less inflammation, and less stress.

If the idea of doing yoga seems overwhelming to you, or your fitness level isn't great, you could start out by doing just a few stretches and/or yoga poses for five to twenty minutes daily. In *Yoga for Cancer: A Guide to Managing Side Effects, Boosting Immunity, and Improving Recovery for Cancer Survivors,* Tari Prinster describes how to create a safe home yoga practice that addresses the different physical needs, risks, and emotions of cancer patients and/or cancer survivors. Her book includes fifty-three yoga poses and twenty practice sequences. These exercises are also beneficial for reducing and managing the side effects of conventional treatments, such as radiation and chemotherapy.[7] So, get out and take a yoga class, buy a yoga DVD, or check out online classes or YouTube videos, and watch the stress melt away as you strengthen your body, mind, and spirit.

Deep Breathing and Meditation

Most of us take breathing for granted and think that because breathing is automatic, we don't need to do anything to breathe better. But most of us breathe in a shallow manner, from our chest rather than our diaphragm, which puts our body into an oxygen-deprived state.

Yet if you take the time to learn how to breathe deeply, it will help you relax and promote your health, as your cells will get more oxygen and you'll find the stress leaving your body with every breath that you take. Not only that, but you'll also be helping your body to directly fight the cancer. Consider this: A 2011 study published in the *Journal of Alternative Complementary Medicine* suggested deep breathing may help reduce the production of free radicals that cause cellular damage, and the practice could also lower blood sugar and insulin levels.[8] High insulin and blood sugar are thought to encourage cancer growth, as do free radicals, so deep breathing can do more than just help you relax; it can help you combat cancer.

Deep Breathing

Deep breathing is easy. Later in this chapter (in the "How to Meditate" section, pages 127–128), I will show you step by step how to do it. If you aren't interested in combining deep breathing with meditation, just ignore the steps in the process that relate to mindfulness.

You can start by practicing deep breathing for just a few minutes daily, to let your body become accustomed to the process. Over time, you'll be able to work your way up to longer periods of time. Once you're familiar with deep breathing, you'll be able to practice it anywhere: at your desk, or while watching TV or making dinner, for instance. This is an easy, free, effective and non-time-consuming stress-reduction technique.

Meditation

In the West, meditation isn't a part of most people's lives. We don't learn about it growing up, and most of us don't think about or practice it until we are faced with a health condition, such as cancer, and our integrative or holistic doctors tell us about it! Yet meditation is one of the most powerful stress-reduction practices there is, not only because it is a calm, quiet activity that you can practice in stillness and solitude, but also because it teaches you how to control your mind and thoughts. And when you can do that, frightening or stressful circumstances can no longer control you. Among its other benefits, meditation lowers high blood pressure and can help reduce symptoms associated with cancer, such as fatigue and pain.

I regularly practice meditation, and when I first began to learn about and practice it, I'll admit—it wasn't easy. But I was so fascinated with it and convinced by its benefits that I decided to stick with it, and not just for myself, but also for my patients' sake. After all, if a practice as safe as meditation can relieve stress and improve your health—all for free, and all without drugs or medications—it is absolutely my duty as a physician to learn about it and then prescribe it.

Many studies have proven the benefits of meditation. One study on 120 women who had received radiation and which was published in 2013 in *Integrative Cancer Therapies,* showed that a program called mindfulness-based stress reduction (MBSR), which combines yoga postures, body awareness, and meditation, improved sixteen variables of the women's health, including certain aspects of physical health and emotional well-being. MBSR also improved the women's ability to cope with the side effects of conventional treatments. Another study of MBSR on women with breast cancer who had received conventional treatment, the results of which were published in 2012 in the *Journal of Clinical Oncology,* suggested similar results. The women experienced an improved quality of life, and better emotional and physical health after practicing meditation for just eight to twelve weeks.

Meditation may seem daunting, but once you get the hang of it, it's actually not that difficult. In this chapter I will show you step by step how to do it (along with diaphragmatic breathing), so you'll be well equipped to incorporate it into your daily wellness regimen.

Meditation is an essential strategy for developing peace of mind. Most of us have millions of thoughts constantly bouncing around in our mind. We need to learn how to slow those thoughts down because a racing mind causes stress. If you have received a cancer diagnosis, you might have a trail of ongoing stressful thoughts, such as: *How am I going to tell my family about my fear of cancer? Why does my belly hurt? Is it serious? Am I going to have to go through this alone?*

We all have a lot to think about nowadays, but it's not good to have your mind turned on all the time and continually processing information that is stressful and difficult, as often happens when you are treating cancer or have just received a cancer diagnosis. Meditation is a great way to break free from the stress of your thoughts and day-to-day life, and learn how to live in greater peace and harmony. In doing so, you'll find that you also feel better in your physical body.

If you decide that meditation is not for you, you can still experience many of its benefits by listening to audio CDs or downloading computer and smartphone-based programs that use special technology to relax you. These programs slow your brainwaves and synchronize your nervous system. In the Resources section, you can find more information on these products.

How to Meditate: At the heart of meditation is a principle called mindfulness. In mindfulness, you take control of your thoughts and basically clear your mind of chaos. It's much like turning down the volume on a blaring radio station until all that you hear is sweet silence. You can do this practice while either sitting or lying down. Meditation also involves deep breathing, while consciously focusing on your breath and allowing nothing into your mind other than the sensations of inhaling and exhaling. Here, step by step, is how to combine deep breathing with mindfulness. If you wish to just do the deep breathing by itself, that is perfectly fine! You will still experience powerful stress-reduction benefits.

1. Lie down on the floor on top of a blanket, and let your back relax into the floor. If that's uncomfortable, try placing a pillow or rolled-up towel under your knees. Keep your shoulders flat and

stretch your torso and neck into a comfortable position. Your chest should be open and your back should feel relaxed and comfortable.

2. Now, focus on inhaling slowly through your nose, while placing your hands on your tummy. As you inhale, make an effort to push your stomach out, instead of your upper chest. Your hands should feel your stomach lifting. This is called diaphragmatic breathing, because you are breathing deeply from the muscle that separates your chest from your abdomen (your diaphragm). In diaphragmatic breathing, your tummy expands and contracts, rather than your lungs. You know that you are doing it right when your stomach expands before your lungs. If, like many people, you are not accustomed to using your diaphragm, this may feel strange or uncomfortable at first. Just give it some time and allow your diaphragm to strengthen. Eventually, belly breathing becomes second nature.

3. After you've filled your lungs, slowly squeeze your stomach back in toward your spine, forcing the air out of your lungs as you exhale. Exhale through your mouth, while focusing on emptying your lungs and compressing your stomach. Ideally, it should take you longer to exhale than inhale. Some people prefer exhaling through their mouth, while others like to exhale through their nose. Personally, I believe that exhaling through the mouth is more effective. Either way, you should hear an audible *whoosh* sound when you exhale. The more air you expel, the more fresh, clean air you'll be filling your lungs with on the next inhale.

Another way to practice mindfulness during meditation is by focusing on an object that brings you joy, such as a beautiful flower or candle, or if you prefer, God. Find a comfortable, quiet place to sit, and then contemplate the flower, or light the candle and watch its flame dance and flicker. During this time, you may notice that your mind becomes distracted by other thoughts. Don't worry, as this is normal in the beginning. Simply acknowledge the thought and let it go, and then focus again upon the object or your breathing patterns.

Meditation and deep breathing take practice, so you may want to start with just a two-minute session and build up from there. Don't expect perfection right away. Getting meditation right isn't a sprint; it's a marathon. Slow, determined, and steady gets you across the finish line and into the winners' circle.

Qigong and Tai Chi

Qigong (which means "energy practice" in Chinese Mandarin) and tai chi are two excellent combination exercise-meditation therapies that promote relaxation and healing by rebalancing the electromagnetic energy of your body though the use of soft, flowing postural movements, focused breathing, and meditation. Tai chi is both a martial art and healing modality (although in the West most people do it for its healing benefits) that originated from a form of Qigong. It is generally thought to be more challenging in its movements and requires more concentration and focus than Qigong, but can nonetheless be a wonderful stress reduction and healing practice.

All of your body's biochemical processes are influenced by energy, so when you balance your energy, you also balance your biochemistry. This is one reason that it's important to not only treat disease on a biochemical level but also the energetic level. Your body's energy flow powerfully affects your well-being.

Both Qigong and tai chi are gentle, unlike some other types of exercise, and are therefore ideal for helping people of nearly all fitness levels to relieve stress, relax their mind, and promote their health. That said, they do require intention and effort, especially tai chi, because concentration and focus are part of the process, but one of the benefits of learning concentration is that it helps you get into the practice of living in the present. Most of us don't do this because we either don't know how, or forget to do so amid our hectic everyday lives.

Qigong and tai chi are becoming increasingly recognized within the integrative medical community in the West for their stress reduction and powerful anticancer benefits. They have been discussed at many recent cancer conferences, although Chinese hieroglyphics suggest that Qigong has been around for as long as seven thousand years, and tai chi since the 1600s.

Qigong may be an easier practice for those with disabilities or who are weak, and Chinese studies suggest it results in improved symptoms in over 95 percent of patients suffering from a wide variety of diseases, including cancer.[9]

In China, Dr. Ming Pang created a type of Qigong practice called Zhineng and set up the largest "medicine-less" hospital in the world, Huaxia Zhineng Qigong Center, where four to six thousand people regularly come to practice Qigong.[10]

The anticancer effects of Qigong and tai chi have been suggested in a number of other studies. Dr. Li-da Feng, professor of immunology at Beijing College of Traditional Chinese Medicine, has done many experiments on external qi (also known as chi, meaning the body's vital internal energy) transmission and claims that a Qigong expert may be able to reduce the incidence of various types of cancer.[11] Similarly, a meta-analysis of thirteen controlled trials on 592 subjects suggested Qigong and tai chi generally improved the subjects' quality of life and immunity, as well as helped reduce their fatigue and high cortisol levels, the latter of which is associated with high stress.[12]

Among their other benefits, Qigong and tai chi may:

- Lower blood pressure
- Increase aerobic capacity
- Improve strength, mobility, and endurance
- Relieve stress and improve nervous system function
- Promote deeper relaxation and better sleep
- Increase immune function
- Improve posture and heal back and spinal conditions
- Clear away negative emotions and reduce anxiety
- Lower stress hormone levels
- Increase the lungs' respiratory capacity
- Increase joint flexibility

If you are ambitious, you can learn Qigong on your own by purchasing DVDs that show you how to do the postures and techniques, or by watching videos online. Or you might find that it's more effective to take a Qigong class in your area. Tai chi may be more difficult to learn on your own, although there are also videos that teach beginner tai chi movements, for those who can't or don't wish to take a class. To find a Qigong or tai chi practitioner, see the Resources section at the end of this book.

Massage

If you don't have the energy or ability to do yoga or Qigong, getting a massage can provide some of the same stress-reduction benefits as these movement-based techniques. Massages relieve stress and anxiety, and stimulate the circulation and movement of lymph throughout your body, which then also helps balance your hormonal and immune systems. It can relieve symptoms of some of the most common symptoms of cancer, including pain, nausea, fatigue, depression, and anxiety. When your body is balanced and you have fewer symptoms, you are generally less stressed.

Studies have also suggested how effective massages can be. One 2005 study published in the *International Journal of Neuroscience* revealed that women who were diagnosed with breast cancer and who received three thirty-minute massages per week were less depressed and angry and had more energy than women with breast cancer who didn't receive massage. Even more significant, the women who had received massage also had an increase in their dopamine levels and natural killer (NK) cell and lymphocyte counts, which are all important cancer-fighting cells.[13]

Some people believe that massage can harm people with cancer, because they fear that it can spread tumor cells, since massage promotes circulation and cancer cells travel through the body via the circulation. But as long as you avoid the tumor area, massage is, in most cases, a safe way to not only relieve stress but also benefit the body.

Surgeon Bernie Siegel, MD, stated, "Massage therapy is not contraindicated in cancer patients; massaging a tumor is, but there is a great deal more to a person than their tumor."[14] So, if you have cancer in an internal organ, you can still receive a comforting and relaxing back, neck, head, or shoulder massage. If you have a tumor and want to work with a massage therapist who understands how to take into account your condition, see the Resources section for information on oncology massage therapists in your area.

Aromatherapy

Aromatherapy is another fantastic tool for lowering stress levels. When you hear the word *aroma*, you might think of inhaling the scent of fragrant candles or a scented lotion, and indeed, many health and household products are marketed as aromatherapy. But true aromatherapy involves using pure plant oils to de-stress and improve the state of the body. These are created from the roots, leaves, seeds, and blossoms of plants, rather than from synthetic chemicals, and can be truly medicinal. Plant oils are believed to have the highest vibrational energy of any substance, and many holistic practitioners believe that when you raise the energy of your body by taking high-energy remedies, you also improve your immune function.

Essential oils are becoming increasingly popular in holistic and integrative medicine, but they are not a new therapy and have been used worldwide to cure disease for nearly six thousand years. The ancient Chinese, Indians, Egyptians, Greeks, and Romans used essential oils medicinally, as well as for many other purposes, such as developing cosmetics, perfumes, and drugs.[15] Among their many benefits, essential oils are widely recognized for their ability to reduce stress, anxiety, and depression, and to alleviate some of the physical symptoms associated with cancer, such as pain and fatigue.

Far from just providing a nice, fragrant scent, aromatherapy is thought to work by causing the smell or nerve receptors in your nose to communicate with the parts of your brain responsible for storing your emotions and memories (the amygdala and hippocampus). When you breathe in the oils, they positively influence your mood. Other researchers think that they promote emotional well-being in other ways, too, such as by interacting with hormones and enzymes that influence neurotransmitters and other bodily chemicals.[16]

You can take plant oils in a variety of ways, in addition to inhaling them. They can be massaged into your skin, or diluted in a vaporizer or diffuser. And unlike candles or other sources of synthetic oils, true essential oils are safe, healthy, and nontoxic, if you use them properly.

Some essential oils that you may want to try for stress relief include frankincense, lavender, rose, orange, bergamot, lemon, and sandalwood. Lavender is especially popular because it is thought to help balance both your physical body and your emotions. Frankincense has a warm, exotic aroma, and along with lavender, is most commonly used to relieve stress, but it also has many physical healing properties as well. Chamomile is a great oil for calming the nerves, and rose is effective for alleviating depression.

Depending on the type of product you purchase, essential oils may need to be diluted with a "carrier" oil, such as coconut, almond, or jojoba, especially if you use them topically. This keeps them from irritating your skin and from you using a too highly concentrated amount of the oil. Nonetheless, it's a good idea to first test any new oil that you use on a small patch of skin inside your wrist to make sure that it doesn't irritate your skin and you aren't allergic to it. Once the oil is diluted, you can rub a few drops of the mixture on your crown, temples, behind your ears, neck, wrists, ankles, over your organs, or on your soles. You can also dilute oils in a vaporizer or diffuser, or place a drop or two on your pillow at night for a more restful night's sleep.

I don't recommend that you ingest essential oils, unless your physician recommends it, as they are very potent when taken this way and can have adverse side effects. I would also advise you to consider consulting with an aromatherapist or other health-care practitioner familiar with essential oils, as some oils can interact with medications and either dilute or potentiate their effects. You'll also want to be careful with essential oils if you have an estrogen-dependent tumor (such as a breast or ovarian tumor) as some oils, such as sage, fennel, and aniseed, contain estrogen-like compounds that can encourage tumor growth. An aromatherapist can help you determine which oils would be most safe and effective for you. To find one in your area, see the Resources section at the end of this book. Many aromatherapists are also trained in other medical disciplines, such as massage or chiropractic. In the Resources, you can also find recommendations for good, pure, pesticide-free essential oil products that can be used for a wide variety of physical and emotional ailments.

Emotional Healing and Stress-Reduction Strategies

So far, we have focused on tools that promote stress reduction through body movements, meditation, relaxation, and similar principles. But when stress is caused by emotional conflicts that require a resolution, sometimes you need a strategy that will help you resolve that conflict, or the thoughts and emotions behind the conflict. The following two therapies, which we and some other practitioners do, are designed to do just that. They can both be done with a practitioner via Skype or over the phone, so you don't even have to leave the comfort of your home to do them.

Recall Healing

Recall Healing was created by holistic wellness expert and consultant Gilbert Renaud, PhD. It is based on the idea that cancer can be caused by what are called "conflict shocks," which are profound emotional conflicts that manifest simultaneously in the psyche, brain, and corresponding organ where the cancer is located. According to the principles of Recall Healing, the brain contains what are called "emotional reflex centers." These centers correspond to different emotions, such as grief, anger, sadness, and so on, which are in turn connected to specific organs in the body. Cancer often develops in the organ or organs that are related to the specific emotional center in the brain that has been affected by the conflict.

Not every emotional conflict leads to disease. Instead, illness occurs only whenever the psychological or emotional conflict that you are dealing with becomes so overwhelming that your psyche, or conscious mind, essentially can't handle it and so downloads, or transfers it into your body. When those conflicts get recognized and resolved, then the state of the body also improves.

With Recall Healing, practitioners can help you discover and eliminate any underlying conflict(s) that may be either causing you to be susceptible to cancer or contributing to it, and assist you in "clearing out" those conflicts from your body and mind. For this process, the Recall Healing practitioner asks you questions about your personal and family history; your thoughts and beliefs, events in your life, and other things that will help him or her discern the root cause of illness.

Recall Healing is very powerful, and many cancer patients I've seen in my clinical experience have said it is the most life-changing therapy that they have ever done. Anyone, with or without cancer, can benefit from this emotional healing process, and usually many conflicts can be resolved within just a session or two of therapy. A few studies have suggested the benefits of Recall Healing. For instance, one Recall Healing practitioner, Michelle LaMasa Schrader, PhD, completed three studies on thirteen people with various health conditions, including cancer, who had used Recall Healing to improve their conditions. Many of the participants reported improved psychological and physical health.[17] To find a practitioner, see www.recallhealing.com and see the Resources section.

The Destination Method (TDM)

The Destination Method (TDM) is a transpersonal coaching and beneficial strategy that I would highly recommend. TDM practitioners, such as creators Robert Dee McDonald, DD, and his wife, Luzette McDonald, DD, see patients in person in a clinical space, but also from the comfort of patients' homes via a Skype or phone consultation.

The Destination Method was developed over fifteen years ago and is based on the premise that our mind—specifically, our thoughts and beliefs—creates our emotional life, which then predictably impacts our physical health. We all create mental "maps," representations of reality that are based on our life's experiences, and which comprise pictures, sounds, tastes, smells, and feelings (based on our five senses).

If you can change your negative mental maps, you will be able to change your emotional state and biochemistry, reduce the stress in your life, and probably see faster healing in your body. TDM teaches you how to do this, and is a quick, effective, and powerful tool for overcoming emotional stressors.

TDM categorizes emotional stressors in the following way:

1. **Shocking images, sounds, or news.** For instance, a cancer diagnosis might cause you to experience shock or trauma. A TDM practitioner might ask you, "What do you see in your mind's eye when you think of cancer?" Often, and understandably, the image may not be very positive, so the TDM practitioner would then help you create a new one that would help you cope during your recovery.
2. **Grief.** Grief often results from the loss of a loved one, although it can also result from losses related to cancer. TDM employs different strategies that can help you resolve grief, such as helping you imagine your lost loved one as being present with you in the here and now.
3. **Traumatic memories.** These are memories that are created by experiences, such as abuse or rape, that occurred recently or long ago. As long as you have traumatic memories, you'll have stress, but TDM can help resolve even this kind of trauma, in just a session or two.
4. **Basic conflicts.** An example of a basic conflict that many people with cancer have is an internal conflict about the desire to get better. For instance, on the one hand, a part of them wants to be healthy—and undeniably so! But in some cases, another part of the patient may not for some reason. TDM can rapidly uncover and resolve such conflicts.

Also, harmful beliefs and behaviors, such as helplessness, hopelessness, and worthlessness, codependence, emotional enmeshment, negative self-talk, unforgiveness, hatred, bitterness, guilt, and shame, can also create thought maps that hinder healing. Maybe you have an "inner critic," a voice that tells you things like "You're stupid" or "You're bad." TDM can help you remove this inner dialogue, or the beliefs that led to the negative inner dialogue, in a short period of time—often after just a single session of therapy.

Unforgiveness is an especially important emotional conflict that TDM seeks to resolve, because you can't have peace and may struggle to get well if you harbor unforgiveness against yourself or others. Dr. McDonald tells his patients that just as gratitude is the foundation of joy, so forgiveness is the foundation of peace. Joy comes immediately when you become grateful, and peace comes when you forgive.

TDM isn't just about choosing to replace your negative thoughts with positive ones, however. Rather, TDM practitioners use techniques for changing your thoughts that are based on thirty different convictions that Dr. McDonald has developed about how the mind works and its relationship to the spirit. TDM is based on the premise that both compassion and precise methods are necessary for improving one's health; TDM practitioners employ an integration of the two.

Let's say that you are suffering from anxiety. According to Dr. McDonald, anxiety is actually worry about the future. It is often linked to the great "What if?" question. For example, you might think, *What if these treatments don't work? What if I can't pay my bills due to my high medical expenses? What if my family abandons me because I'm so sick?*

But anxiety isn't about circumstances as much as it is about the things that you see in your "mind's eye" and what you say to yourself in your "mind's ear." For instance, if you tell yourself that your cancer diagnosis is horrible, and that you're going to end up sick, abandoned, and alone, those thoughts tend to create anxiety. Similarly, if you think you're depressed because you were just diagnosed with cancer, the depression isn't about the diagnosis as much as it is about your internal dialogue and your beliefs about cancer, rather than your circumstances.

Or maybe you believe that the future is hopeless, because you are helpless to change the undesirable or difficult circumstances of your life. Such beliefs have been founded upon things that you have experienced in the past or present through your five senses—through images that you have seen in your "mind's eye," or what you have heard through your "mind's ear" and so on, but which are not necessarily truth or reality, but rather, your perceptions of reality.

Of course, many of us suffer from emotional conditions, such as anxiety and depression due to biochemical factors; say, a deficiency of serotonin caused by illness, or low thyroid function, in which case we also believe that it's important to treat those underlying biochemical imbalances. On the other hand, resolving the cognitive causes of anxiety, depression, or other harmful emotions can often help change our chemistry, and vice versa.

We have found TDM to be very effective for helping reduce our patients' anxiety and stress levels, often after just one session. You can learn more about TDM and get a practitioner referral at the TDM website. See the Resources section for more information.

Journaling

Journaling is another great emotional healing and stress-reduction strategy that you can do from the comfort of your home and which doesn't cost anything but a bit of your time. Journaling involves writing down your thoughts and feelings, the events of your day, or your goals. It can help you process, unload, and sort out the challenges of cancer, identify things in your life that you appreciate or want to change, or discover emotional issues that you may need to heal. If you don't like to write, you can also sketch and draw pictures as a way to process or express your emotions and thoughts.

Research has suggested that journaling may help people experience a greater sense of emotional well-being and even physical healing. For instance, in one study, a group of early-stage breast cancer patients were asked to either write their deepest thoughts and feelings about breast cancer, or focus on the positive things that had happened to them during their experience with cancer. After several months, the women who did this had fewer symptoms and medical appointments than women in another group who had been asked to simply report the facts about their treatment.[18]

Journaling is a worthwhile stress-reduction strategy, especially if you find that you don't have the time or money to pursue the other healing solutions that are described in this chapter. This is because journaling for even fifteen minutes daily can help you release pent-up emotions and get clarity on your future plans or issues that might be concerning you.

Finally, consider sharing your challenges with a close friend as well as on paper. This can sometimes be just as therapeutic as the other healing solutions described in this chapter, and it costs nothing. We all need to be able to share and process our struggles, and friendships are one great way to do that.

Make Humor and Laughter a Part of Your Day

This is a simple strategy for stress reduction, but you'd be surprised at how many people neglect to laugh. Find a sitcom to watch on TV, get a funny book to read, or look for humorous anecdotes on the Internet—basically, anything that will get you to smile! Or simply spend more time with your friends and family members who love to laugh.

Humor and laughter are powerful medicine, especially during stressful times. Laughter helps minimize stress by boosting immunity, increasing pain tolerance, and minimizing the negative elements of the stress response. A 2013 study suggested, for instance, that laughter increased the immune function of people with gastric and/or colorectal cancer.[19] Learning to laugh, which may seem tough when you're dealing with a cancer diagnosis, really is good medicine.

Nightly Hot Bath

Finally, consider taking a hot bath every night to relieve your tension and stress. A hot bath relaxes your muscles, can help reduce the pain of tension headaches, and promotes circulation. Taking some time to be alone in the bathtub to read a good book, pray, or meditate can also help you relax by taking your mind off of the worries of the day, and give you a break from the hectic pace of your daily life.

You can enhance the physical and emotional benefits of a bath by lighting candles and placing them alongside the edge of the tub, or by adding a drop or two of pure lavender oil, or Epsom or Celtic salts, to the water. These calm your nervous system, and are a cheap way to detoxify your body and help your muscles relax. You can also make an aromatherapy bath using mineral bath salts. See the Resources section for some high-quality calming aromatherapy bath products.

SUPER STRESS-REDUCTION STRATEGIES		
Strategy	What It Is	Major Benefits
Yoga	A physical and spiritual discipline that uses a combination of postures, rhythmic breathing, and meditation to reduce stress and promote health in the body	• Increases energy, strength, and flexibility • Improves circulation and oxygenates the body • Relieves pain • Detoxifies the body • Stimulates immune function • Produces peace and relaxation
Deep Breathing	Breathing slowly, deliberately and purposefully from the diaphragm, or the belly, rather than the lungs.	• Reduces stress and anxiety • Oxygenates the body and reduces the production of free radicals that cause cellular damage. • Can reduce symptoms associated with cancer
Meditation	Practicing "mindfulness": taking control of your thoughts and clearing your mind of chaos. Often used in combination with deep breathing.	• Reduces stress, anxiety, and depression • Oxygenates the body when combined with deep breathing

continues

SUPER STRESS-REDUCTION STRATEGIES   continued

Strategy	What It Is	Major Benefits
Qigong/Tai Chi	Combined exercise-meditation therapies that promote relaxation and healing by rebalancing the electromagnetic energy of the body though the use of soft, flowing postural movements, breathing, and meditation. Tai chi is generally thought to require more concentration and to be more challenging than Qigong in its movements.	• Increases aerobic capacity • Improves strength, mobility, and endurance • Relieves stress and improves nervous system function • Promotes deeper relaxation and better sleep • Increases immune function • Improves posture and heals back and spinal conditions • Clears away negative emotions and reduces anxiety • Lowers stress hormone levels
Massage	Using gentle hand movements to massage the back and other areas of the body	• Relieves stress and anxiety • Stimulates circulation and the movement of lymph • Balances the hormonal and immune systems • Can also relieve common symptoms of cancer, especially pain and fatigue
Aromatherapy	Inhaling or topically applying pure, medicinal plant oils to the body. Oils are created from the roots, leaves, seeds, and blossoms of plants.	• Reduces stress, anxiety, and depression • Can relieve physical symptoms of many conditions, including pain and fatigue

Emotional Healing and Stress-Reduction Strategies

Strategy	What It Is	Major Benefits
Recall Healing	A technique for discovering emotional conflicts that contribute to disease and resolving those with a RC practitioner	• Resolves emotional conflicts that may be causing or contributing to cancer (www.recallhealing.com)
The Destination Method (TDM)	A technique for discovering how and what negative "mental maps" are affecting your thoughts, emotions, and body	• Helps you create healthier "mental maps," thoughts, and positive emotions that foster health (www.teloscenter.com)
Journaling	Sharing your thoughts and emotions, events of the day, and goals on paper	• Helps you process, unload, and sort out the challenges of cancer; identify things in your life that you appreciate or want to change; or discover emotional issues that you may need to heal.
Make humor and laughter a part of your day	Laughter, telling jokes, watching funny shows/movies	• Releases stress and promotes joy • Promotes immune function
Nightly hot bath	Immersion in hot water. Best done with Epsom salt or aromatherapy oils.	• Relieves stress and anxiety • Relaxes the muscles • Detoxifies the body • Improves circulation

EMILY'S Story

After I was diagnosed with stage 2 uterine cancer in 2011, I decided to pursue natural remedies for treating it. About a month after my diagnosis, I scheduled my first appointment with Dr. Connealy. She and I shared a lot of the same philosophies about what would work for me. We both knew I needed to reduce the stress in my life and detoxify my body, and that I needed an herbal protocol to help the cancer leave my body. She also reminded me about many great stress-reduction tools that I'd used before but which had fallen to the back burner of my mind, and reinforced the importance of me using them.

One great stress-reduction tool that I used along the way was yoga. I didn't have a lot of energy at the time, so I would do gentle exercises and take a class so that I would feel like a normal human participating in life.

I also used humor to elevate my mood so that I wouldn't get down about having to take a lot of supplements. I told my friends a lot of humorous stories to keep my mood light and to help me recognize that the bout with cancer wasn't my whole life but just a chapter in it.

Finally, another powerful tool that I used was meditation, which I continue to use as my daily time to connect with God or the divine, because I knew that God was part of my healing team and process. So, my mantra in the morning during meditation was, "God before technology," and my philosophy was, "Sit down before you boot up." This is so important because the mind, especially when you are ill, will take you to some very terrible places. I would get into the habit of meditating first thing in the morning before I would even look at my phone or turn on my computer. Through meditation, I could observe where my mind wanted to go—which was usually "hell"—and then bring it back to where I wanted it to go and change my thoughts in a way that would facilitate my healing.

CHAPTER 9

Strengthen Your Immune System with Sleep

IN THIS CHAPTER, YOU WILL LEARN . . .

- How getting a restful night's sleep protects and helps beat cancer
- The causes of insomnia or poor sleep
- Solutions for sound sleep, including proper sleep hygiene and supplements

A significant number of cancer patients say they don't sleep well. And they are not alone. A poll by the National Sleep Foundation found that more than half of all Americans between the ages of thirteen and sixty-four rarely or never get a good night's sleep, and about two thirds (63%) say their sleep needs aren't met during the week.[1] Clearly, we have an epidemic of insomnia and related sleep difficulties in this country.

Yet getting a quality night's sleep, all night, every night, isn't just a luxury; it is critical to your health, metabolism, immune function, and in readying you to take on the next day. Deep, restful sleep gives your body a chance to renew and repair damaged cells. When that process is interrupted, health problems become inevitable. In fact, research suggests insufficient sleep is even more harmful to your health than a lack of exercise.

During the different stages of sleep, your body is doing anything but resting. It's repairing muscles and tissues that have been damaged throughout the day; releasing hormones that regulate aging and appetite, storing your memories, recharging your brain, and boosting your energy supply. These unconscious activities affect every aspect of your physical and mental health, and have a tremendous impact upon your quality of life. So, whenever you don't get enough sleep, you may find yourself suffering from a wide variety of symptoms, including brain fog, poor concentration, anxiety, sore muscles and body aches, increased appetite, weight gain, and recurring bouts of colds and the flu. Studies have also suggested that people who don't get enough sleep may be at an increased risk for cancer, for many reasons.

How Poor Sleep May Promote Cancer

When you don't sleep, your body produces fewer natural killer (NK) cells and less melatonin. If you'll recall from Chapters 6 and 7, NK cells are one of your body's frontline immune defense against cancer, and melatonin has cytotoxic effects against it. Sleep deprivation also raises inflammation and cortisol levels, and causes insulin resistance and weight gain, which are all risk factors for cancer. What's more, a whole series of detoxification pro-cesses occurs when you sleep. If you don't sleep well, you will often feel horrible, and accumulated toxins don't get removed from your body but instead continue to damage your cells, causing yet another potential setup for cancer.

Many studies have drawn a link between sleep deprivation and cancer. One study showed that insufficient sleep might contribute to breast cancer recurrences among postmenopausal women and the development of more aggressive forms of breast cancer.[2] Another study suggests that disrupted sleep increases prostate cancer risk.[3]

If you are unsure whether you are sleeping well, and you have a nighttime sleep partner, consider asking him or her, "How do I sleep?" You may be waking up periodically throughout the night or snoring and keeping your partner awake, unbeknownst to you.

To live a cancer-free life, you must get your beauty rest! Many factors can cause you to be sleep-deprived. Next, I describe some of the most common (and commonly overlooked) ones, as well as solutions that aim to help you get better rest.

Causes of Insomnia

Stress

Stress, either short- or long-term, can cause poor sleep. When you are stressed, or you find your mind filled with racing thoughts or on "fast forward" before bedtime, try listening to relaxing music or meditative audio. You can also download meditation programs onto your smartphone or computer. Some audio programs, such as Centerpointe Research Institute's Holosync, can help you clear the chaos from your mind by slowing your brain waves into a meditative, or low-frequency, state by using a special auditory technology. Other programs utilize guided imagery and cognitive techniques to induce relaxation. Some, such as Heart Math technology, also track your heart rate variability (HRV) on your smartphone so you can see whether you are effectively getting into a relaxed state. For more information on these products, see the Resources section at the end of this book.

If you don't want to invest in stress-reduction technologies, you can practice some of the stress-reduction techniques described in Chapter 8, such as deep breathing, meditation, and aromatherapy before bedtime. Or you might try taking a stress-reducing supplement, such as Phosphatidyl-Serine, which can help lower cortisol levels that contribute to late-night wakefulness. For information on recommended products, see the Resources section.

Sleep Apnea

Sleep apnea afflicts an estimated 28 million Americans. This is a condition in which you either have pauses in your breathing or stop breathing for short periods throughout the night. There are two main types of apnea: central and obstructive. Central sleep apnea happens when your nervous system fails to activate your breathing muscles during sleep. Obstructive sleep apnea occurs when your airway collapses or is blocked during sleep.

A 2015 analysis of two independent studies associated sleep apnea with higher cancer incidence and premature death.[4] This is probably because oxygen, which we know helps fight cancer, does not get to the apnea sufferer's tissues and organs as easily or as much as it should.

If you wake up exhausted, your partner tells you that you snore, or you are exhausted and sleepy during the day, you may have apnea. You can do a test, either at home or in a sleep study clinic, to find out if you have this correctable condition. The American Academy of Sleep Medicine, for instance, has sleep testing centers nationwide (see the Resources for more information). If you find that you have apnea and it is mild (and depending on the cause), you may be able to treat it by avoiding sleeping in certain positions, such as on your back; by avoiding taking sleep medications and alcohol; and if you are overweight, by losing weight.

If the apnea is more severe, your doctor may recommend CPAP therapy. "CPAP" stands for "continuous positive airway pressure." For this, you wear a mask over your nose and/or mouth at night, while a machine delivers a continuous flow of air into your nose. The airflow keeps your airways open so your breathing stays regular. CPAP is the most common treatment for sleep apnea.

Depending on the cause of the apnea, you may also benefit from a special type of dental device that will keep your airway open during sleep, and which is designed by biological dentists who have special expertise in sleep apnea. For more information about where to find a good biological dentist, refer to the Resources section.

Lack of Exercise

Lack of exercise is a common cause of restless nights, because your body discharges stress hormones during exercise that would otherwise keep you awake at night. But the only exercise that some of us get is to move between an office chair and a car seat or bed! As a result, stress hormones accumulate in our body and make it difficult for us to sleep.

Research supports the idea that doing exercise can improve our sleep. For instance, one study showed that Qigong (described in Chapter 8)—a Chinese practice that typically involves meditation, coordinated slow movements, and deep rhythmic breathing—improves sleep and reduces symptoms of fatigue and depression.[5] For some examples of exercises that you can do, no matter your fitness level, see Chapter 7.

Poor Nutrition

Eating junk food or foods that you're allergic to creates inflammation in your body, which can prevent you from getting deep, restful sleep. You may also suffer from insomnia if you don't get all the right kinds or amounts of vitamins and minerals in your food or supplements because nutrients are involved in sleep processes. For example, magnesium plays an important role in sleep, but magnesium deficiency is common among those who eat the Standard American Diet (SAD). Magnesium deficiency is also related to other conditions that cause insomnia, such as restless leg syndrome, anxiety, and tense muscles.

Medications

If you're taking a medication and have trouble sleeping, check with your doctor to find out whether insomnia is a potential side effect of that medication. Everyone reacts differently to medications, so even if you know other people who are taking the same prescription as you and they are sleeping well, that same medication could still be a problem for you. Also, while sleep medications and antidepressants may help you sleep better in the short term, they could worsen insomnia in the long run because they cause your body to more rapidly use up its supplies of serotonin and other mood- and sleep-enhancing neurotransmitters. They can also cause other serious long-term side effects, such as memory loss, a rapid heartbeat, dizziness, dry mouth, depression, moodiness, constipation, and restlessness, just to name a few. Finally, sleep medications can decrease your body's production of GcMAF, which is the main director of your immune system. If you are taking this sort of medication, I recommend consulting with your doctor to make sure that they aren't interfering with your immune function.

Hormone and Neurotransmitter Imbalances

Many of us have hormonal imbalances due to stress; environmental toxins, such as plastics and electromagnetic fields; illness; a nutrient-deficient food supply; aging; and other factors. These imbalances manifest themselves in such conditions as PMS, thyroid problems, metabolic syndrome, diabetes, and adrenal insufficiency. They cause a wide range of symptoms, from fatigue to depression, headaches, weight gain, and, you guessed it—insomnia.

Hypothyroidism, or low thyroid function, for instance, can cause insomnia, as can estrogen dominance, a condition in which you have too many harmful chemicals in your body that mimic the actions of estrogen. Both hypothyroidism and estrogen dominance are common in our society. Even adrenal fatigue, which results from chronic, unrelenting stress and is often referred to as "burnout syndrome," creates an imbalance in important hormones, such as cortisol, DHEA, and pregnenolone, and can alter sleep in a number of ways. If you have adrenal fatigue, you might have blood-sugar regulation problems that cause you to have episodes of low blood sugar during the night. Your body then awakens you to alert you that you need food. Or your body's natural cortisol rhythms might become inverted so that you are tired during the day and awake at night. Similarly, neurotransmitter imbalances or deficiencies, such as low serotonin or GABA, or excessively high levels of excitatory neurotransmitters, such as epinephrine and glutamate, can keep you awake at night.

It is beyond the scope of this book to describe in detail how imbalances of all of your body's chemicals can disrupt sleep, but you may want to get your hormones and neurotransmitters tested by a reputable lab if the other sleep strategies described in this chapter don't help you get the shut-eye that you need. See the Resources section for more information.

Most skilled integrative doctors do hormone and neurotransmitter testing. If your doctor doesn't do saliva or urine hormone or neurotransmitter testing, you may be able to find one in your area that does by doing a practitioner search on the American College for Advancement in Medicine website, acam.org.

You can often treat hormone and neurotransmitter imbalances by making simple dietary and lifestyle changes, and doing regular detoxification therapies. At other times, you may also need to take supplemental nutrients or bioidentical hormones. For more information on hormone and neurotransmitter balancing, I recommend reading *Why Isn't My Brain Working?* by Datis Kharrazian, DHSc, DC, MS.

Other Causes of Insomnia/Poor Sleep

Other common causes of insomnia or poor sleep include electromagnetic pollution, caffeine, and alcohol. Take alcohol, for instance. The notion that having an alcoholic beverage in the evening encourages relaxation or sleep is actually misleading. You may find that a drink relaxes you, but even one drink can disrupt your sleep patterns, if you are sensitive. One clinical study found that when people consumed alcohol within an hour of bedtime, they fell asleep more easily, but the alcohol then disrupted their sleep later in the night.[6]

Similarly, caffeine disrupts sleep by stimulating the nervous system. Caffeine's effects on the body last for about eight hours, so drinking a cup of coffee after lunch, around one p.m., can disrupt your sleep at night. Also, such beverages as noncola sodas, chocolate, and so-called natural energy drinks sometimes contain caffeine. If you must have food or beverages containing caffeine, consume them only in the morning.

Finally, electromagnetic pollution is becoming an increasingly important reason that many of us are suffering sleep loss and walking around like zombies. You can reduce the EMFs in your sleep environment by unplugging any appliances in your bedroom, and/or turning off your circuit breakers at night; turning off your cell phone, and unplugging your Wi-Fi connection, all of which generate high levels of EMFs.

Solutions for Sound Sleep

There are many things you can do to overcome insomnia or fitful slumber in addition to the strategies I've mentioned so far. In the following sections, I share some of these.

Practicing Proper Sleep Hygiene

One of the most important things that you'll want to do to get good, deep, uninterrupted shut-eye is create an environment that's conducive to rest. This may sound obvious, but you'd be surprised at how many people don't do this. Here are some tips for creating your sleep sanctuary.

First, darken your bedroom as much as possible. Your body will stop producing melatonin, a crucial sleep hormone, if there is even a small sliver of light coming in through your bedroom window. So, unplug any glowing gadgets, dim the lighting on your digital alarm clock if possible, and make sure to use blackout curtains on your windows if you sleep past dawn or have outdoor lamps shining into your bedroom. If you can't darken your room sufficiently, consider purchasing some eyeshades, and if you are sensitive to noise, use earplugs.

Second, get to bed at a reasonable time. In a culture of 24/7 everything, it's easy to overlook the fact that our body is designed to be active in the daylight and rest when it's dark. It's ideal to get to bed by ten p.m. because your body produces the most melatonin and removes toxins most effectively between ten p.m. and two a.m. So, if you don't go to bed until one a.m. or nod off while the TV is on, getting eight hours of sleep is not going to make up for the fact that you've missed out on the prime melatonin-producing portion of the night.

Other things you can do to prepare your body for sleep include doing relaxing activities at night, such as taking a hot Epsom salt bath, turning off your computer at least a couple of hours before bedtime; having a cup of chamomile tea, and making sure not to exercise within two hours of bedtime.

Sleep Supplements

Mother Nature has provided us with a pantry full of herbs that have helped people sleep for centuries. Some of my favorites include valerian, hops, lemon balm, chamomile, passionflower, and lavender. These herbs relax the nervous system, are safe, and don't cause side effects in most people. Occasionally, some people might experience headaches or early morning sluggishness the morning after taking them, especially if they are taken at higher doses. Their use may also be contraindicated if you are taking certain medications, especially those with sedative properties, so I recommend first consulting your doctor to determine whether they are appropriate for you. All of these herbs can be taken in capsule form, or you can make a tea from them before bedtime. You can find them at most health food stores as well as at many online retailers.

Amino acids, such as 5-HTP, L-tryptophan, and GABA can also relieve insomnia or restless sleep. They are especially useful if you have brain chemistry imbalances. Your body uses 5-HTP to make a neurotransmitter called serotonin, which regulates your sleep, mood, energy, and other functions. Available in capsule form, 5-HTP can be purchased online or over the counter at health food stores. Try taking one or two 100 mg capsules of 5-HTP thirty minutes before bedtime. If you are sensitive to supplements, you may want to start with just one 50 mg capsule to see whether that is enough and then gradually increase the dosage to 100 to 200 mg. L-tryptophan, which is a precursor to 5-HTP, is also a great amino acid that is a powerful adjunct and/or substitute for 5-HTP. Some people get better results by taking 5-HTP; others, by taking L-tryptophan; and still others, by taking both types of amino acids, so you may want to experiment to find out which one works best for you. If you decide to try L-tryptophan, start with just one 500 mg capsule thirty minutes before bedtime. See the Resources for product and additional dosing recommendations.

While it is safe for most people to take these amino acids, they may be contraindicated in certain situations. For instance, if you are on antidepressant medication, you'll want to consult your doctor before taking 5-HTP or L-tryptophan, since they affect serotonin levels, as do most antidepressant medications.

GABA is a calming amino acid and neurotransmitter that can also be tremendously beneficial for sleep, if 5-HTP or L-tryptophan don't do the trick. Start out with one 250 mg capsule thirty minutes before bedtime, and if that doesn't work, increase to two capsules, or 500 mg. I like to think of GABA as "natural Valium" because it is a natural sedative. Like the other amino acids, GABA may be contraindicated for some people or in certain situations, such as if you are taking sleep or other medications that have sedative properties, so you'll want to consult your doctor before taking it if you are on these types of medications. Also, overdosing on any amino acid can cause dangerous side effects, so start with the lowest recommended dose, and be sure to consult your doctor to confirm that you are on the right dose. For information on recommended amino acid products, see the Resources.

Over fifty percent of the population has a methylation problem, or a defect in a gene called MTHFR, which helps the body make neurotransmitters from amino acids. If this is you, then your body will not be able to make and utilize amino acids very well, and you will feel poorly whenever you take them, or they simply won't work well for you. You can find out whether you have a MTHFR gene mutation by doing a simple test, called "MTHFR," through your local lab. A properly functioning MTHFR gene is absolutely essential for the proper functioning of many metabolic pathways, not just neurotransmitter synthesis, so it's a good idea to find out whether this gene is working well.

If you discover that it isn't, you can take nutrients to help your body properly create neurotransmitters from amino acids. The most common and effective of these include methyl B_{12}, which is a certain type of vitamin B_{12}; L-methylfolate, SAMe, and P5P. P5P is a bioavailable form of vitamin B_6 that your body can readily use.

The particular type and amount of nutrients you'll need, as well as the dosage, will depend on your test results. Or you could try experimenting with a small amount of methylfolate, or P5P, to see if you feel better when you take amino acids or they seem to work better in your body.

Melatonin

Melatonin is a hormone made by your pineal gland, which is a pea-size gland located in the middle of your brain. During the day, this gland is inactive, but at night and in the presence of darkness, it produces melatonin, which enables you to sleep through the night. Nowadays, many of us don't produce sufficient amounts of melatonin because we are exposed to factors that inhibit its release, such as bright light from lamps, computers, and smartphones late at night. Many studies support this idea. For instance, a 2011 study published in the *Journal of Clinical Endocrinology and Metabolism* suggested that exposure to room light in the late evening not only suppresses the amount of melatonin that is produced in the body but also reduces the amount of time it remains in the body by about ninety minutes.[7] So, if you are exposing yourself to bright light later in the evening, you may be shortening your body's melatonin cycle by an hour and a half, and getting fewer hours of deep, restful sleep at night.

You'll want to avoid bright light before bedtime, but you may also benefit from taking supplemental melatonin to help increase your body's natural melatonin levels and restore your sleep-wake cycle. Melatonin can be purchased at most health food and grocery stores, and is the only hormone that is legally sold over the counter. It's a good idea to consult your doctor when determining how much to take, as too-high doses can actually interrupt sleep, and may be contraindicated in certain conditions (see Chapter 6). In general, though, melatonin is a safe supplement. You can find melatonin product recommendations in the Resources section.

From my clinical experience, most patients find that they are able to sleep by practicing the sleep hygiene strategies and/or taking the supplements recommended in this chapter. Occasionally though, and as a last resort, we may need to prescribe them sleep medication. I usually prescribe trazodone, which is technically an antidepressant but also works well for sleep. I prefer to avoid prescribing medications, but it's much better for people to get the restorative rest that they need than for them to not sleep. So, when all else fails, you may want to ask your doctor for a prescription of trazodone or another nonaddictive sleep medication.

SLEEP SOLUTIONS	BENEFITS
Practicing good sleep hygiene Examples: • Darkening the bedroom at night • Unplugging glowing gadgets/TV • Using earplugs/face mask • Going to bed by ten p.m. • Taking a hot bath (with Epsom salt) • Not using the computer or exercising within two hours of bedtime	• Creates a quiet, dark environment and puts your body into a state of relaxation. Also restores your sleep-wake cycle.
Audio CDs and other downloadable sleep technology	• Brings your body, especially your brain, into a state of deep relaxation
Supplements	
Herbal remedies Examples: valerian, chamomile, hops, lavender, lemon balm, passionflower	• Contain sedative properties that relax your brain and body
5-HTP	• Promotes serotonin production, which plays a role in sleep and mood (among other functions) Dosage: 100–300 mg before bedtime
L-tryptophan	• Promotes serotonin production, which plays a role in sleep and mood Dosage: 500–1,500 mg before bedtime
GABA	• Balances GABA, a calming neurotransmitter that acts like a natural sedative and induces sleep Dosage: 500 mg 1–3x/night
Melatonin	• Regulates your sleep-wake cycle • Has anticancer properties Dosage: 1–3 mg before bedtime

RICK'S Story

I've been doing treatments for bladder cancer with Dr. Connealy for about a year and a half, and she has always said to me how important it is to get enough sleep. For most of my forty-year career, I was a respiratory care practitioner, and would work nights and sleep only five hours a day, so my sleep rhythms weren't normal. I'd come home from work and go to bed around seven a.m. and then get up by noon, and head back to work at six p.m. I did this for many years and often relied on lots of caffeine to keep me going. I'd also notice that the night-shift nurses whom I worked with were generally tired and had a tendency to put on weight. Even I noticed that I was starting to get a belly by the end of my career, and I had always been a slim person.

Since I no longer work nights and now sleep seven or eight hours, my outlook on life has dramatically improved. I have more energy and no longer feel like I'm missing out on life. In addition, I practice good sleep hygiene, don't eat or drink within three hours of bedtime, and get to bed by eleven p.m. I have also since cut out coffee and drink green tea instead, and believe that I sleep a bit better because I am no longer being constantly stimulated and am not as amped up all day.

I'm doing well now; all of my cancer test markers are low, and I wake up in the morning with a smile on my face.

PART THREE

THE CANCER REVOLUTION PLAN
FOR HEALTH AND WELLNESS

Putting Together Your Support System

When you're diagnosed with cancer, you want to be armed and equipped with four essential survival tools, including:

- Knowledge about treatments, both traditional and integrative
- The right team of health-care practitioners
- An advocate, helper, or "cheerleader"
- A mind-body-spirit treatment plan

Putting Together a Successful Support System

Knowledge is power: You'll want to start your wellness journey by educating yourself about all of the different available treatment options and doctors. No two integrative cancer doctors are alike, and not all will offer exactly the same menu of tools or services. That's why I would encourage you to find a doctor or team of doctors that use many of the cutting-edge and evidence-based tools described in *The Cancer Revolution*, or similar ones. You can research doctors and their approaches at the following medical association websites:

- Academy for Comprehensive Integrative Medicine: www.acim connect.com.
- American College for Advancement in Medicine: www.acam.org
- International Organization of Integrative Cancer Physicians: www .ioicp.com.

So, for instance, you might go to acam.org, click on the "Resources" link, and then the "Physician+Link" tab. You would choose the "oncology" option to look for cancer doctors, compile a list from the results, and then go to the physicians' websites to study their treatments. Especially research those doctors who have a long list of treatments in their toolbox because you will want to address your cancer treatment from as many angles as possible.

Once you have compiled a list of doctors, call them and interview them and their staff. Don't be shy! This is your life, and it's important that you get the best care that you can. Get lots of opinions so you are well informed, and have an idea about who and what's out there. Don't make an appointment with just anyone and hope for the best.

As you talk with the doctors and their staff members, ask yourself which ones resonate with you and what you need. Pay attention to whether they listen to you. Notice whether they value your input, and whether they seem to be positive and encouraging, because you want your support system to be comprised of positive, uplifting people who care about your feelings and opinions.

You'll also want to communicate with former patients of the doctors whom you interview if possible. One way to do this is by asking around on large Internet cancer forums about others' experiences with those particular doctors. Alternatively, you might give your name and phone number and other information to the prospective doctors' staff, to pass along to former patients who might be willing to share their experiences with that doctor. Do as much research as you can; study the doctors' websites, talk with their staff, and learn as much as possible before entrusting your wellness regimen to them.

As part of your interview process, you might ask your prospective doctors the following:

1. **What factors do you base your treatment regimens on?**
   A successful regimen will never be based upon just the cancer itself but rather, the totality of what's going on in your body. A well-informed and wise doctor will analyze the intricacies of your body and create a regimen that's based on your personal needs rather than give you a cookie-cutter, one-size-fits-all protocol.

2. **Do you prepare a specific diet plan for each patient and tailor it to their unique needs?**
   You want to find a doctor who will create a detailed, unique food plan for you based on your lab findings.

3. **Do you include detoxification, stress reduction, and other mind-body-spirit healing tools in your regimens?**
   If the doctor only focuses on cancer treatments, look elsewhere to find another who understands a whole-body approach and that other things are as just as crucial to your recovery.

4. **Do you continually educate yourself about the latest discoveries in medicine and about how the human body works?**
   You want to find out whether the doctors whom you are interviewing are content with the status quo or the established standard of care.

5. **Do you utilize innovative new techniques and treatments on an ongoing basis?**
   Every doctor should do this! Medical knowledge doubles every two years, so doctors who are serious about helping their patients overcome cancer need to stay abreast of all the newest and best wellness tools and cutting-edge scientific strategies—both in conventional and integrative medicine—and continually use them in their practice.

6. **Are you knowledgeable about both conventional and alternative treatments?**
   A well-informed and successful cancer doctor should understand conventional oncology as well as all the available alternative, natural, and complementary therapies, and how to effectively combine them. They shouldn't have a bias toward a particular type of medicine—because both chemotherapy and natural treatments

have their place in cancer treatment—but should instead understand the pros and cons of each type of medicine, and what *you* will need at each stage in your wellness process. There is a precise timing and an art to prescribing medicines and therapies, and successful physicians know what therapies to combine, when, and how.

Finding a doctor has become easier in recent years, as many integrative cancer doctors can do long-distance consults via Skype or telephone. So, if you can't find a good doctor in your area, consider meeting with one in another state or even another country. Some doctors who do Skype may first require an initial consultation in person, but others will not. Most testing and lab work can also be done long distance.

There are advantages to seeing a physician in person, such as being able to receive a hands-on examination and do more on-site therapies, but many integrative doctors can get a pretty good idea about what patients need simply by talking to them and having them do tests. That said, in my clinical experience, I have always advised cancer patients to do an initial consultation with their new integrative doctor in person because it establishes a stronger rapport, a positive connection, and a more solid relationship overall. If it's not possible for you to do a face-to-face, in-person meeting, the next best thing is a live Skype video chat. So, don't feel that just because you live in a remote location, you can't get good cancer treatment. You have options!

You may also find that you need multiple health-care practitioners on your team. In addition to your integrative doctor, these might include any, some, or all of the following:

- **A conventional oncologist** because it's important that cancer patients be aware of all of their treatment options
- **A nutritionist** if your integrative doctor isn't very knowledgeable about anticancer food plans
- **A counselor or minister** to help you to navigate the emotional aspects of your recovery
- **A physical therapist or trainer** to help strengthen your body, especially if you are weak and not ambulatory

Once you have decided upon a doctor or team of health-care practitioners, and you feel confident that they are a good fit for you, determine to fully follow their recommendations. Of course, if along the way something doesn't seem to be working out, you should always let your doctor(s) know, because you want to be fully on board with your plan and content with the doctor or practitioners you have chosen to be on your team. If you aren't, and over time, you start to have doubts about them or your treatments, then you'll want to either resolve your concerns with them or find a different doctor or practitioner.

Finding an Advocate, Helper, or "Cheerleader"

Many cancer patients find that, between the stress of being ill and the side effects of some treatments, they have difficulty doing things, or remembering instructions and details. Some of patients, for instance, may have memory problems, or don't know how to read and follow instructions. They may have cognitive problems that prevent them from doing this or other things, or they may not be fully committed to getting well.

If this is you, then you'll want to find an advocate, helper, or "cheerleader": a family member, companion, ally, or friend whom you trust to be an ambassador for you and who can do such things as accompany you to your doctors' appointments, prepare your meals, help you organize and follow your treatment regimen, and sort through your treatment options, as well as support you emotionally. This person should be someone who can inspire you when you are down, encourage you, and simply be there for you in case you need a helping hand or moral support.

You might think that just because you aren't in a wheelchair or are functional enough to work, you don't need help. But the truth is, cancer is a challenging, life-changing illness that can be difficult to navigate on your own, and most everyone, no matter how strong or optimistic, needs a shoulder to lean on, an ear to talk to, or a voice of inspiration in their midst. This can be especially true during the initial stages of diagnosis and treatment when you are still trying to figure things out and establish a new routine.

Don't be shy about asking for help—you might be surprised to find that some people will consider it an honor and a privilege to participate in your recovery. For instance, we have found that some of our patients' co-workers will give up their sick leave or vacation days for them. It may be hard for you to ask for help because perhaps you were raised to believe that you're just supposed to "pull yourself up by your own bootstraps." Or maybe deep down, you just don't believe that you are worth it.

Regardless, we aren't meant to get by in life on our own, so if this is you, I encourage you to reach out to others despite your discomfort because you deserve to get well, and when you are well, you can more effectively help other people. The ancient expression "It takes a village" was originally coined to mean that it takes an entire community of people to raise a healthy child, but it also applies to battling cancer; I strongly believe that the more support you have around you, the smoother and better your road to recovery will be.

If you're not sure how to ask for help, one strategy might be to create a support letter to send to your friends, family, and co-workers. Tell them you have been diagnosed with cancer and you want to invite them to participate in your recovery process. Include a list of your needs: what you need help with, when, why, and how. These needs may include:

- Rides to the doctor's office
- A secretary who can take notes for you during your appointments. (It can be difficult for some people, especially those who have had chemotherapy and who might have "chemo" brain, or brain fog, to remember doctors' instructions or take adequate notes.)
- Help with shopping
- Cleaning house
- Organizing supplements and/or putting together an at-home treatment plan
- Preparing meals for the week
- Providing a listening ear or companionship
- Financial donations for treatments/living expenses

After you have compiled your list and your letter, tell your contacts it would mean a lot to you if they could help you with one or more of the tasks on the list. You could also send the letter to the pastor or leader of your local church, synagogue, or other membership association that you belong to. Faith or humanitarian-based organizations that help others as part of their mission may be especially willing and able to help you.

If you don't have anyone around to help you, no friends or family members, or volunteers at your local church, club, or other place of membership, consider seeking paid help for at-home care or counseling. If you have limited funds, you could set up a fund-raiser on such websites as www.GoFundMe .com. These sites are becoming an increasingly popular way for people with fewer resources to raise money for treatments, home health care, and more.

Just be sure to check out these websites' terms and services pages to be fully aware of any tax implications for funds raised on the site and to ensure that your cause is approved for their use.

Consider also connecting with others through an in-person or online support group for people with cancer. Such groups often provide a tremendous source of emotional support, as well as resources and insights into how to deal with the day-to-day difficulties of cancer. You can find a wide variety of cancer support groups online. Yahoo! Groups is one great option for this. See the Resources for more information.

Unfortunately, many insurance companies do not cover unconventional cancer tests or natural and integrative treatments. I like to think integrative clinics practice "tomorrow's medicine," but most insurance companies have not yet caught up and do not cover a lot of what several integrative doctors do. A limited number of insurance companies may pay for office visits, routine blood work, physical therapy, and preventive care, but it depends upon the company. Yet one advantage of integrative treatments is they tend to be less costly than conventional treatments, and whether patients choose integrative or conventional therapy, they still end up spending a lot of money out of pocket in either case.

LOU ANN'S Story

In February 2014, I was diagnosed with stage 2 breast cancer. I had a lumpectomy to remove the tumor, but also decided to go to the Cancer Center for Healing to do other treatments.

I have made amazing progress. In July 2014, she did a CTC blood test on me, and by then, my numbers had already gone down to from 6.8 to 3.8. In November 2014, I had a breast MRI, which came out clear. And in May 2015, I had an ultrasound and everything also came out clear on that.

I've had a lot of support, in addition to my doctors and nutritionist, which has helped me tremendously in my healing process. First, I came up with the idea to start my own support group, and I decided that it would be a group that would give people hope (as well as me), and it has been really healing for everyone. In the last group meeting, for instance, we discussed gratitude, and how important it is to be grateful, even when you are going through a cancer diagnosis. We need to be thankful for the valleys as well as the mountaintops. There's a reason that everyone gets cancer, and sometimes it can be a blessing in disguise. Having this attitude has really changed my life.

The people at my church have also been very supportive. My priest anointed me in the presence of my family and friends before my surgery. He often asks how I'm doing, and has continued to keep me in his prayers. Also, a group of girlfriends from my church started a group called "The Wholiness Plan," which involves meeting once a week in each other's homes to share healthy recipes, pray, and support one another.

Last but not least, my family and friends have really supported me, but I had to first tell them, "As I go through this journey, I want you to know that I am not going to go the conventional route of treatment. I know that this might be hard for you to accept, but I only need positive reinforcement right now (which means accepting my decision to do integrative medicine)." So they, including my husband, were very supportive and positive. I could always feel the effects of their prayers, especially when I went in for surgery to remove the tumor, because I was surrounded by peace.

Finally, I don't think that I would have been as strong or healed so quickly and completely without the help of Jesus Christ, my Lord and Savior. In fact, my faith has been the most important thing to me throughout this process. As the Bible says, "I can do all things through Christ who strengthens me" (Phil 4:13, NKJV).

CHAPTER 11

Creating an Anticancer Living Environment

IN THIS CHAPTER, YOU WILL LEARN . . .

- How to detect and remove toxins, such as mold, EMF pollution, and other contaminants from your home environment
- How to choose nontoxic household and personal care products for optimal wellness

Once you have put together your wellness team and are armed and ready with a solid treatment plan, the next thing you'll want to do is turn your home into a toxin-free sanctuary that promotes recovery. I tell my patients, "We don't live in a petri dish" (a pristine environment of controlled conditions). Our environment is more like a goldfish bowl that needs to be cleaned regularly and kept clean and free of toxins. Because what happens if you never change the water in your goldfish bowl? The goldfish can become sick or die.

To prevent or heal from cancer, you can't just eliminate the cancer-causing toxins from your body; you'll need to get them out of your home and ideally your work environment as well. A clean home is part of the recipe for wellness and you can't just skip this part of the recipe. You will undermine your treatments, healthy diet, and detoxification efforts if you do.

We simply don't live the same way that people did one hundred years ago, before there were thousands of electromagnetic and chemical toxins in the environment. The world we currently live in is inhospitable to the survival of humans, and integrative doctors know that because we are seeing the rates of all kinds of disease, from autoimmune illnesses to cancer, autism, and heart disease, skyrocket in recent years. Cancer was once a disease reserved for the old, but nowadays, it isn't uncommon to see children and young adults who have been diagnosed with cancer. We can't be indifferent and look the other way anymore if we want to survive and thrive as a species, so we all need to do our part and remove every source of toxicity that we can from our environment, if only for the sake of our own safety and wellness. Most of us can't make our homes perfect, but there is a lot that you can do to clean up your "goldfish bowl." And you don't have to do everything all at once; changing your environment little by little can go a long way toward helping you in your battle against cancer or in helping you remain well.

Detoxify Your Home

Personal Care and Household Cleaning Products

If your home is like most people's, it's likely to be filled with potentially toxic, chemical DNA-damaging household cleaning and personal care products. Most laundry and dish soaps; floor, carpet and bathroom cleaners; and other household cleaning products are replete with chemicals linked to cancer, such as:

- **Perchloroethylene, a.k.a. perc.** This potentially toxic chemical solvent is used to dry-clean clothes, draperies, bedding, and curtains. One way to help avoid exposure to this component is to instead take curtains, bedding, drapes, and clothes that are labeled "dry-clean only" to a "wet cleaner," which uses water-based technology, such as liquid carbon dioxide (CO_2), rather than chemical solvents to clean fabrics.
- **Ammonia.** This is found in many household cleaning products. You can determine whether a product contains harmful ammonia or ammonium compounds by doing a search on the Environmental Working Group website (www.ewg.org) and typing "ammonia" into the search engine box. The site will pull up a list of products that contain ammonia and rate them from A to F. A rating of D or F means that the product contains ingredients that are potentially

significant hazards to the environment (and your health). Instead, make your own products, using natural substances, such as vinegar, tea tree oil, and baking soda. They work just as well! You can find natural, nontoxic cleaning product recipes for every household need on a variety of online websites, such as Eartheasy.com. See the Resources section for more information.

- **Chlorine.** This is found in many bathroom cleaning products, as well as in tap water. Use natural substances and products, such as Bon Ami, borax powder, hydrogen peroxide, vinegar, essential oils, and baking soda to clean your bathrooms instead. I like to mix a few drops of an essential oil, such as orange or lemon, into a gallon of water, along with a splash of vinegar and hydrogen peroxide. For detailed information about how to make your own bathroom cleaning products using these and other substances, see the Eartheasy website. See the Resources for more information.
- **Triclosan.** This phenol ether derivative is found in most liquid dishwashing detergents and hand soaps. Instead, choose from among the abundance of natural dishwashing, laundry, and dishwasher soaps on the market, such as those made by Seventh Generation and Mrs. Meyer's.

These are just a sampling of the most toxic cancer-causing chemicals found in most household cleaning products, but you don't need to memorize the names of all the different toxic ingredients that are out there. As a rule of thumb, if a product has a perfumed or chemical smell, or ingredients on the label that you can't pronounce, there's a greater chance the product contains toxic ingredients. Similarly, most personal care products, such as deodorant, shampoo, soap, body lotion, and cosmetics, also contain chemicals that some research has linked to cancer and other diseases. Some of the most common chemicals in these products include:

- Phthalates
- Parabens
- Mineral oil
- Petrolatum
- Propylene glycol
- Sodium lauryl (or laureth) sulfate

- FD&C color pigments (which are made from coal tar)
- Fragrance (a euphemism that could mean anything; note that such products as Mrs. Meyer's use natural essential oils for scent)
- Triclosan
- Aluminum (a toxin commonly found in antiperspirants)

Research suggests an association between exposure to these chemicals and cancer. For instance, a 2013 study published in the *Journal of Inorganic Biochemistry* suggested that high concentrations of aluminum in the breast (usually caused by aluminum-containing antiperspirants) cause oxidative damage to the cells and inflammation, both conditions that lead to cancer.[1]

With personal care products, it can be more difficult to recognize whether a particular product is truly healthy for you because many "natural" or "organic" products contain a combination of both harmful chemicals and natural ingredients. So, consider compiling a list of commonly used toxic ingredients in personal care and beauty products, and take that to the store with you when you shop, and read product labels. Or, better yet, research products by name at the Environmental Working Group site, which contains a database that rates the safety of over seventy-two thousand household, personal care, and cosmetic products. See the Resources section for more information.

Believe it or not, the skin ingests these types of chemicals and assimilates them into your body. The great news is there is an abundance of excellent natural replacements for cancer-linked cleaning and personal care products. Some large grocery stores carry at least a few all-natural cleaning and personal care products, but you're likely to find a wider selection at your local health food store or online. See the Resources section for household cleaning product recommendations.

If you wear makeup, you'll also want to choose natural mineral makeup over mass-market makeup, which typically contains a long list of questionable substances, many of which are banned in other countries outside the United States. Again, refer to the Resources section for a list of excellent personal care and beauty products. Visit the Environmental Working Group site for even more ideas.

Cookware

You can eat healthy, organic food, follow your food plan to a T, and detoxify your body daily, but if you cook and store your food in the wrong kinds of pots, pans, and dishes, you may be undermining your efforts to keep your body clean and toxin-free. Many types of cookware contain heavy metals and other chemicals associated with cancer that leech into the food whenever you heat or store food in them. These include pots, pans, and storage containers made from plastic or from aluminum and certain other types of metal. Avoid Teflon and other nonstick coatings as well. Experiments conducted by the Environmental Working Group have suggested that when Teflon-coated pans are heated, their plastic coating breaks apart and emits toxic chemicals. These chemicals can be lethal to pet birds and may cause a variety of illnesses in humans, including cancer.[2]

While cookware can be expensive, it's best if you can replace your toxic pots and pans with ceramic, cast-iron, or glass cookware. Stainless-steel products are acceptable if they don't contain a high amount of other metals, such as nickel. You can determine the quality of your stainless-steel products by placing a magnet inside them. If the magnet sticks to them, they are likely to be safe. If it doesn't, then that suggests there are a high percentage of undesirable metals in the cookware, in addition to the stainless steel, so you don't want to use it.

Along these same lines, make sure to also store your food in glass or ceramic, rather than plastic containers, which may leech phthalates into food. As discussed, phthalates are also linked to cancer. That said, also aim to choose waxed paper over plastic wrap.

Other kitchen appliances that you'll want to consider replacing with less toxic options include your microwave, deep fryer, and BBQ grill. Deep fryers and grills cook foods at high temperatures, and in so doing, remove the healthy enzymes from them. Cooking at high temperatures also creates cancer-causing free radicals that damage the body. A 2012 study published in *Food Chemistry* suggested that when three different types of oil were heated to a frying temperature of 190°F, cancer-linked compounds called aldehydes were formed.[3] You may also want to consider getting rid of any electrical appliances whose food and/or liquid-touching elements are made of hard plastic. Coffeemakers are among the most common of these. Instead, choose a stainless-steel coffeemaker or water kettle, both of which tend to be made with less hard plastic.

Finally, microwaves emit cancer-linked radiation that, at high doses, has the potential to damage and alter the configuration of food. They also project potentially damaging radiation into the kitchen or room that the oven is in. While little research has been conducted specifically on microwave ovens, according to Joseph Mercola, DO, on his site Mercola.com, "Standing a foot away from it [the microwave] while it's running can expose you to upwards of 400 milliGauss of radiation, and a mere 4 milliGauss has been firmly linked (in studies) to leukemia."[4]

The safest and healthiest way to cook your food is by sautéing, steaming, baking, or broiling.

Carpeting, Linens, and Other Household Items

Once you've exchanged all of your potentially toxic chemical personal care products, as well as traded your household cleaning products and cookware for nontoxic natural ones, the next thing you'll want to do is consider the composition of your carpet and home furnishings. I realize that you may not be able to just run out and buy new furniture if they are composed of cancer-linked materials, but as you read the following section, consider whether you might have a mattress, rug, or something else in your home that is triggering your allergies, making you tired, or otherwise causing you to feel less than your best. If so, you'll want to exchange that item for a healthier version.

Your carpet may contain various cancer-linked chemicals, such as formaldehyde, as well as mold spores, dust, and bacteria, which aerosolize into the air and then get into your lungs when you breathe. New carpet particularly is laden with chemicals. Fortunately, you can now find nontoxic carpet from such companies as Nature's Carpet and EarthWeave, which make carpeting from all-natural wool, a material that actually helps clean, rather than contaminate, the air. See the Resources section for more information.

Alternatively, if you are able, you may want to consider exchanging your carpeting for hardwood, natural stone, and/or tile flooring. If you can't do this, consider purchasing a HEPA or propolis air filter to help mop up airborne toxins that either come from or end up in the carpet. Remember, the air inside of your home is far more toxic than the air outside, even if you live in a big city, so it's worthwhile to invest in an air filter.

Toxic mattresses and bedding may also cause problems, but like all things described in this chapter, there are excellent natural replacements for them. If you have a conventional mattress (especially a new one), chances are it contains petroleum-based polyester, nylon, and/or polyurethane (PU) foam, all of which can emit volatile organic compounds (VOCs) into the environment, which are linked to cancer. Most mattresses are also treated with flame-retardant (FR) chemicals, which may be toxic. Additionally, the metal springs in most mattresses can be hazardous to your health, because they conduct with electromagnetic fields (EMFs) in the environment and may amplify the effects of EMFs upon your body. So, if you suspect that your bed is making you sick, or you just want to make sure that it isn't, consider replacing your mattress with an all-natural one made from 100% wool, organic cotton, or natural latex. Similarly, choose 100% organic cotton sheets, pillowcases, and other bedding; likewise, 100% organic cotton toweling and rugs for your bathrooms.

VOCs are also found in building materials, chemical cleaning products, paint, solvents, carpet, vinyl flooring, air fresheners, and photocopiers, among other things. You can't eliminate every source of VOCs from your environment, but here are some things that you can do to reduce your exposure to VOCs in your home:

- Avoid purchasing conventionally treated mattresses brand new.
- Open windows throughout your home on a daily basis (as the weather permits).
- Avoid purchasing new carpet if you have health problems (because all new carpet contains high levels of VOCs).
- Use natural household cleaning products.
- Use low-VOC paint for your household painting projects. (This can be found in most home improvement stores.)

Again, you don't have to do everything all at once, but you want to reduce your toxic burden as much as possible, and little by little. The sicker or more immunity-compromised you are, the more important that this will be.

Other Household Toxins

Mold

Mold may be one of the most dangerous toxins linked to cancer, and yet it is found in as many as half of all households across the United States and worldwide, and especially in damp climates. According to toxin expert Lee Cowden, MD, "The mycotoxins [mold toxins] produced by mold are more toxic and harmful to the body than any other manmade toxin except for some radioactive elements."[5] And mold specialist Ritchie Shoemaker, MD, contends that approximately 25 percent of all people can't effectively remove mold toxins from their body.[6]

Sometimes mold is visible and you can see it. At other times, it is invisible and hiding behind your walls or washing machine, or perhaps under your bathroom or kitchen sink. If you have a leak somewhere, such as around your bathroom shower or toilet, or behind your washing machine or dishwasher, and the floor or wall around that area feels cold to the touch, then this means that there may be mold there.

Not all types of mold are toxic, but if your home smells musty, you have a water leak, or live in a damp climate, you may want to order a simple, do-it-yourself mold test called ERMI (Environmental Relative Moldiness Index), which looks for the presence of more than three dozen harmful mold species in your home. It does this by analyzing a sample of dust from your carpet. You can order a testing kit online; see the Resources section for more information.

If you discover through the ERMI test that you have a dangerous type of mold in your home, it's critical that you get it removed by a professional mold remediator. You'll then want to ask your integrative doctor to test you to find out whether that mold is causing you symptoms or negatively affecting your immune system and compromising your recovery. There are things that you can do to detoxify your body from mold, but it's not a do-it-yourself treatment; you'll want to enlist your integrative medical doctor to help you.

Clean Up Your Air

Studies suggest indoor air is more polluted than outdoor air, so I highly recommend getting an air purifier for your home and/or workplace. This will reduce the amount of toxic burden that your body has to deal with, so that it can focus on keeping you healthy, or aiding your cancer battle. Some great air purifiers include those made by Austin Air. These remove such things as dust, hair, pet dander, mold, pollen, chemicals, gases, and odors from the environment. Alternatively, if you can't afford these types of air purifiers, which can average $500 or more, you can purchase a propolis air vaporizer or diffuser, which uses a component of beehives, to help sanitize the environment. Propolis has been proven to eliminate germs, mold, and some other types of pollutants from the air. One company that makes these diffusers is Bee Healthy Farms. For information on where to get these air filters, see the Resources.

If you are on a tight budget, you can do a lot to clean up your air just by opening some windows in your house during the day, or by getting a few plants. Plants clean up the air by absorbing harmful gases, such as carbon dioxide, benzene (found in some plastics, fabrics, pesticides, and cigarette smoke), and formaldehyde (found in chemical dish detergents, fabric softeners, and carpet cleaners).

Electromagnetic Pollution

Electromagnetic pollution is potentially one of the most dangerous household toxins to which we are all exposed. We discussed electromagnetic pollution in Chapters 5 and 9, along with some suggestions for reducing electromagnetic fields (EMFs), especially in your sleep environment. In addition to the solutions shared in those chapters, you may want to also unplug any appliances when you aren't using them; use wired communications in your home, such as a landline for your phone, and a hardwired Internet connection for your computer (instead of Wi-Fi and cordless phones). Consider purchasing Graham-Stetzer filters, to protect you from EMFs that come through the wall wiring and your smart meter. If you live within 600 feet of a power line or microwave tower, you may want to consider painting your walls with EMF-protective paint or even moving. Refer to the Resources for information on where to purchase EMF-protective products for your home.

Detox Your Life

The following table summarizes some of the most important things that you'll want to do to clean up your food, water, air, and home, as discussed in this and previous chapters. Use this table to do a fast check of whether you are on track with most of the detoxification recommendations described in this chapter and throughout this book. Most of us forget aspects of our treatment regimen from time to time, so this table can help remind you of those things that you might have a tendency to forget or that you want to address at a later time.

TIPS FOR CLEANING UP YOUR AIR, WATER, FOOD, AND HOME	
Air	• Avoid smoking or being in an environment of secondhand smoke. • Use a high-quality HEPA and/or propolis air purifier in your home and/or workplace.
Water	• Use a reverse osmosis water filter for your kitchen sink and/or the rest of your home, or purchase a Berkey water filter or alkalinizing water products by pH Prescription Water (www.phprescription.com), pHenomenal water (www.pHenomenalwater.com) and Purative.com. Use an Aquasana filter for your shower.

continues

TIPS FOR CLEANING UP YOUR AIR, WATER, FOOD, AND HOME continued

Food	• Consume only organic fruits and vegetables (grown without pesticides, herbicides, and other synthetic fertilizers). • Buy fruits and vegetables fresh. Frozen produce is acceptable when fresh isn't available. • Consume only grass-fed, hormone- and antibiotic-free meat. Try US Wellness Meats (www.grasslandbeef.com) for quality animal protein products. • Eat smaller fish low in mercury and heavy metals, such as wild salmon and sardines. Avoid tuna, swordfish, shark, king mackerel, red snapper, orange roughy, moon fish, bass, marlin, and trout, which have high mercury levels. Try Vital Choice Seafood (www.vitalchoice.com) for high-quality wild salmon and other fish. • Wash all vegetables with vinegar or a veggie wash spray. • Consider a ketogenic or other low-carb diet, or a healthy vegetarian/vegan diet. • Avoid processed foods with artificial preservatives, including all cured foods. • Avoid foods and beverages that contain sugar substitutes, such as aspartame (NutraSweet and Equal). • Avoid all refined sugar, which is cancer-causing. Choose stevia as a healthy substitute. • Avoid most grains, dairy products, alcohol, and caffeine, and any other allergenic foods.
Food preparation & storage	• Drink water out of glass or stainless-steel jars or cups, instead of plastic bottles. • Store and cook your food in stainless-steel, glass, or ceramic containers. • Broil, bake, steam, or sauté foods. • Buy lunchmeat wrapped in waxed paper rather than plastic, and condiments in glass. • Bag your groceries in paper rather than plastic. • Avoid aluminum, plastic, and nonstock materials, such as Teflon. • Avoid frying, microwaving, and barbecuing foods. • Avoid heating food in plastic containers or with plastic wrap over the top. • Avoid canned foods and foods stored in plastic.
Household & personal care products	• Choose natural household cleaning and personal care products made by such companies as Dr. Bronner's (www.drbronner.com), Mrs. Meyer's (www.MrsMeyers.com), and Organic TKO (www.tkoorange.com). • Choose natural makeup, made by such companies as Osmosis (www.OsmosisSkinCare.com) and Eminence (www.EminenceOrganics.com). • Eliminate all synthetic chemical personal care, household building, repair, and cleaning products, and replace with natural ones. • Avoid perfumes and air fresheners that contain benzene, aluminum, and other cancer-causing chemicals.
Medication & nutritional supplements	• Find natural alternatives to birth control pills, blood pressure medications, antidepressants, synthetic hormones, and other medications. • Choose natural and bioidentical hormones over synthetic ones. • Avoid taking antibiotics except in an emergency. • If you use prescription drugs, make sure that you understand their potential side effects and long-term complications.

continues

TIPS FOR CLEANING UP YOUR AIR, WATER, FOOD, AND HOME continued	

Do-it-yourself detoxification tools	• Do regular detoxification therapies daily. These include:
	  • Sauna
	  • Coffee enema and/or liver flush
	  • Epsom salt bath
	  • Juicing
	  • Taking toxin binders, such as zeolite
	  • Rebounding
	  • Body brushing
	  • Walking
	• Exercise regularly and moderately to remove toxins.
	• Get out in the sun, but avoid excessive exposure to sunlight.

JO ANN'S Story

In 2012, three years after my divorce, I was diagnosed with stage I breast cancer. I believe that the stress that I experienced in my marriage is part of what caused the cancer. The conventional approach to medicine wasn't enough, and it didn't address my immune system, so in the fall of 2012, I began to pursue healing with Dr. Connealy and the Cancer Center for Healing. She had me do such things as IV vitamin C and heavy metal chelation, and prescribed melatonin and trazodone for sleep since my battle with breast cancer and the treatments had affected my ability to sleep. She also put me on some other supplements, including a product called MAP from Germany, which helped me rebuild muscle tissue after my surgery. I am now free of breast cancer, but I have to do things to stay well, and I watch myself carefully.

As part of this, and because my son has an autoimmune disease, I try to keep toxins out of our home. Unfortunately, we live in a world where there are a lot of toxins in the environment that are making people sick. So, for instance, I drink alkaline water (Kangen brand) and have done so since 2009, to try to keep my body as alkaline as I can. I use Mrs. Meyer's organic, natural laundry and dish soap. I also don't use the old aluminum-based deodorants. Instead, I use a brand called Tom's of Maine. Because I've had mercury toxicity, I take toxin binders, and do other detox therapies, such as colonics and infrared saunas. I also use pharmaceutical-grade skin cleanser. I'm still trying to switch over to organic makeup, but I haven't yet found a brand that I really like.

To clean up my home, I got a new bed and pillows that are made of organic materials, and I am trying to find a carpet and padding that don't outgas toxic substances. So, I'm trying to do as much as I can without being a fanatic about it. My family calls me the "woo-woo" sister, but I try to pass on as much helpful information as I can to my family, anyway, because I know it's important.

CHAPTER 12

The 14-Day Anticancer Wellness Plan

IN THIS CHAPTER, YOU WILL LEARN . . .

- How to put together everything that you've learned into a personalized 14-day plan
- How to create a food plan using your recipes and MAP supplements
- How to measure your ketones and calculate food portions on a ketogenic or other low-carb food plan
- Essential anticancer "superfoods" that you should incorporate into your meals

---

You're likely overwhelmed with trying to manage your cancer battle, so this chapter will provide you with a straightforward, easy-to-follow roadmap that includes all the wellness tools and strategies described in this book that you can do at home. It focuses on the six key factors for health discussed in Part 2—a healthy food plan, detoxification, supplements, exercise, stress reduction and emotional well-being, and sleep—and how you can include them in your daily regimen.

Your cancer treatments are not included in the plan because you will be working with your doctors and support system to formulate your treatment regimen; however, you'll definitely want to share the 14-day plan with your doctor to make sure it is appropriate and beneficial for you, and doesn't

174

counteract or contradict any of his or her recommendations or treatments. He or she may want to modify the plan to better fit your needs.

You may notice that some of the practices in the 14-day plan will enable you to address multiple aspects of your regimen at once. For instance, exercise isn't just useful for detoxifying your body, but also for reducing stress and improving your mood—all at the same time. Meditation reduces stress, enhances your emotional well-being, and improves your sleep. Epsom salt baths help you detoxify, reduce stress, and sleep.

Feel free to add other practices or substitute the suggested activities and/or tools for others that better suit your needs, or do them at a time of day that works better for you. For instance, I have placed your daily exercise program and coffee enemas in the morning, but you could do these things after breakfast, or lunch, or dinner. Just avoid exercising too close to your bedtime, or you may not be able to sleep well at night.

At the end of the 14-day plan is a chart you can use to fill in your daily activities and custom-tailor the plan to your needs. For example, I have not specified a supplement regimen in the plan because everyone's supplement schedule will be different, so you can use the chart to add supplements to your daily regimen. The only supplements I have included in the plan are the Master Amino Acid Pattern (MAP) supplements. I introduced these in Chapter 4, as they are part of your diet. (Note: You can also substitute Perfect Amino by Body Health for MAP supplements. For more information, see Chapter 4 and the Resources.) The following is more detailed information about MAP.

MAP Supplements

MAP supplements are a great substitute for animal protein in your meals because unlike when you consume animal protein, your body generates virtually no nitrogen waste when you take them and they are 99 percent bioavailable, or usable, by your body. The nitrogen waste that our body makes when we eat animal protein puts a strain on our kidneys and liver. By reducing your intake of animal protein and taking MAP supplements, you can detoxify and repair your body more effectively, and keep your acidity and waste levels low.

When taking MAP, start slowly, with just two capsules, twice daily, thirty minutes before meals. Then, increase the amount gradually until you reach your desired dosage, which could be up to ten capsules, two or three times daily. Once you reach that dosage, consider replacing the animal protein in your lunch or dinner once or twice weekly with MAP, optionally increasing the evening dose to six to ten capsules and eliminating animal protein from your evening meal. It is best to take MAP during your evening meal, to give your body a more extended break from having to digest animal protein. The following is a suggested dosing schedule for MAP, but you'll want to consult with your physician to help establish dosages that are most appropriate for you. Dosing is generally based upon body weight. So, for example, a person who weighs 90 to 130 pounds may want to take 5 or 6 capsules, twice daily; a person who weighs 130 to 150 pounds, 7 or 8 capsules, twice daily; and a person who weighs more than 160 pounds may want to take 8 to 10 capsules, twice daily. For this reason, the MAP schedule in the 14-day plan is simply a guideline. You'll want to adjust it to fit your needs.

Suggested MAP Dosing Schedule

> Monday and Tuesday—2 MAP capsules, twice daily
> Wednesday and Thursday—3 MAP capsules, twice daily
> Friday and Saturday—4 MAP capsules, twice daily
> Sunday and Monday—5 MAP capsules, 2 to 3 times daily
> Monday and Tuesday—5 MAP capsules, twice daily, and so on.

The Cancer Revolution 14-Day Plan

The 14-day plan includes many of the meals that you'll find in the Recipes section at the end of *The Cancer Revolution*, as well as ideas for meals and snacks that are so simple to prepare that you don't need a recipe. The recipes listed here are suitable for most people who are on a ketogenic or other low-carb, anticancer diet (more information on the specifics of the ketogenic diet can be found on page 199 as well as in Chapter 4). However, as noted in Chapter 4, people have different carbohydrate needs on the ketogenic diet, which means the following plan may or may not put you into ketosis, so that your body burns fat rather than glucose for energy. You may need fewer carbohydrate-containing foods or in lesser amounts than what are contained in the 14-day plan meals, or you may be able to tolerate more carbohydrates and still remain in ketosis. If your doctor believes that a ketogenic diet is best for you, you will want to work with him or her to determine the exact amount of carbohydrates that you'll need for your body to go into ketosis.

Above all, the 14-day plan is meant to provide sample anticancer meals that emphasize fewer carbohydrate-containing foods and higher amounts of healthy fats and protein. It is ideal for helping you prevent or fight cancer, regardless of whether it puts you into ketosis because it is low in carbohydrates and healthy, but you'll want to work with your doctor to refine and adjust the plan according to your particular needs.

If you are not on a ketogenic diet and your doctor recommends that you follow a higher-carbohydrate or other type of food plan, that's okay—it is likely that you can still use many, if not most, of the following recipes in the 14-day plan. Or you may just need to make small adjustments to the meals, such as adding more vegetables or fruit, or consuming fewer protein-based foods. The portions outlined in this plan are simply recommendations. If you are athletic or male, for instance, you may be able to have larger meat or protein portions; up to 6 ounces per meal.

As a final note, I recommend consuming fresh wheatgrass daily as part of the 14-day plan. You can prepare fresh wheatgrass using a wheatgrass extractor or purchase ready-made wheatgrass from your local health food store. It is best to consume 2 to 4 ounces of pure wheatgrass daily, but you can also prepare a Mega Greens wheatgrass powder drink (see Resources for product information) by mixing a scoop of Mega Greens powder with 8 ounces of purified water in the morning, which will aid in detoxification and bowel cleansing. (Note: Fresh wheatgrass is generally safe to consume, but if you have severely compromised immune function, it's best to consult your doctor before taking it, as fresh wheatgrass can occasionally contain mold or bacteria.)

Week 1, Day 1

WHEN YOU WAKE UP

Do oil pulling for 5 to 20 minutes (see Chapter 5 for instructions on oil pulling), to remove any toxins that have accumulated in your bloodstream during the night. Then, if you have time, take a tongue scraper and brush your tongue to remove any fungi, bacteria, and dead cells from the surface. This will give your immune system a quick boost in the morning and help prevent any fungal overgrowth in your body.

BEFORE BREAKFAST

Drink 8 to 16 ounces of lemon or vinegar water, and/or take 2 ounces of fresh wheatgrass. Alternatively, prepare a Mega Greens Drink in 8 ounces of purified water (page 230).

Do a coffee enema.

Take 2 MAP (Master Amino Acid Pattern) capsules, 30 minutes before breakfast.

Do 30 minutes of yoga, Qigong, stretching, walking, or another exercise.

Do 30 minutes of meditation, journaling, or prayer, to start your day off right and more effectively stave off stress during the day.

BREAKFAST

Whey or Plant Protein Powder Drink (page 233)

SNACK (OPTIONAL)

1 ounce or 1 to 2 slices of nitrate-free turkey luncheon meat with 1 to 2 tablespoons of Fresh Guacamole (page 240)

30 MINUTES BEFORE LUNCH

8 ounces of high-quality alkaline water

2 MAP capsules

LUNCH

1 (4- to 6-ounce) Ground Chicken Patty (with Lettuce Wrap) (page 276), 1 tablespoon of Spicy Burger Sauce (page 239), 1 cup of sliced cucumber

MIDAFTERNOON

2 ounces of wheatgrass or 8 ounces of Mega Greens Drink (page 230)

15- to 30-minute walk, stretch, rebounding, or other movement activity (according to your fitness level and schedule)

SNACK (OPTIONAL)

½ cup of Cinnamon Chia Pudding (page 282)

DINNER

3 to 5 ounces of Herb Almond Crusted Mahimahi (page 274), 1½ cups of Fennel with Turmeric (page 269)

BEFORE BEDTIME

1 cup of Fiber Drink (page 235) or herbal tea

Coffee enema (if you did not do this in the morning), sauna, and/or body
  brushing. (Note: Doing coffee enemas at night may cause wakefulness
  in some people, so I generally recommend doing them in the morning.)

Journaling, meditation, or prayer (if you didn't do this in the morning)

For sleep: aromatherapy or Epsom salt bath, sleep audio, herbal supplements,
  melatonin, and/or amino acids

Week 1, Day 2

WHEN YOU WAKE UP

Oil pulling and tongue scraping (optional)

BEFORE BREAKFAST

Lemon water and/or 2 ounces of fresh wheatgrass or 8 ounces of Mega Greens
  Drink (page 230)

Coffee enema

30 minutes before meal, take 2 MAP capsules

30 minutes of walking, yoga, Qigong, or stretching

30 minutes of meditation, journaling, or prayer

BREAKFAST

2 to 3 Poached Eggs (page 236) or Hard-Boiled Eggs (page 236), 2 slices of
  Turkey Bacon (page 237), ½ avocado

MIDMORNING

8 ounces of Iced Green Tea (page 234) and/or 2 ounces of fresh wheatgrass
  or 8 ounces of Mega Greens Drink (page 230)

30 MINUTES BEFORE LUNCH

8 ounces of lemon water

2 MAP capsules

LUNCH
3 to 5 ounces of Garlic Lemon Dijon Chicken (page 274), 2 cups of Baby
      Greens Side Salad (page 253), 1 tablespoon of Citrus Delight Dressing
      (page 250)

MIDAFTERNOON
Mega Greens Drink (page 230)
15- to 30-minute walk, stretch, rebounding, or other exercise/activity

SNACK
1 cup of herbal tea, 1 celery stick with almond butter

30 MINUTES BEFORE DINNER
8 ounces of purified water
2 MAP capsules

DINNER
3 to 6 ounces of Garlic Herbed Shrimp (page 278), 2 cups of Arugula Side
      Salad (page 253) or Baby Greens Side Salad (page 253), 1 tablespoon
      of MCT Essential Salad Dressing (page 249)

BEFORE BEDTIME
1 cup of Fiber Drink (page 235) or herbal tea
Epsom bath, sauna, and/or body brushing
Journaling, meditation, or prayer (if you didn't do in the morning)
For sleep: aromatherapy or Epsom salt baths; sleep audio, herbal supple-
      ments, melatonin, and/or amino acids

Week 1, Day 3

WHEN YOU WAKE UP
Tongue scraping and oil pulling (optional)

BEFORE BREAKFAST
Lemon water and/or Simply Greens Detox Beverage (page 228)
Coffee enema
3 MAP capsules
30 minutes of yoga, Qigong, stretching, or walking
30 minutes of meditation, journaling, or prayer

BREAKFAST
Coco Loco Nut Shake (page 233)

MIDMORNING
2 ounces of fresh wheatgrass or 8 ounces of Mega Greens Drink (page 230)
3 MAP capsules

LUNCH
1 cup of Hearty Beef Soup (page 264), 2 cups of Baby Greens Side Salad
   (page 253), 1 tablespoon of Citrus Delight Dressing (page 250)

SNACK
1 Hard-Boiled Egg (page 236) or 1 cup of Savory Sipping Alkaline Broth
   (page 235)

MIDAFTERNOON
Mega Greens Drink (page 230)
3 MAP capsules
15- to 30-minute walk, stretching, rebounding, or other exercise/activity

DINNER
3 to 6 ounces of Baby Rack of Lamb (page 272), 2 cups of Kale Side Salad
   (page 253), 1 tablespoon of MCT Essential Salad Dressing (page 249)
Chamomile tea

BEFORE BEDTIME
Fiber Drink (page 235)
Epsom bath, sauna, and/or body brushing
Journaling, meditation, or prayer (if you didn't do in the morning)
For sleep: aromatherapy or Epsom salt bath, sleep audio, herbal supplements,
   melatonin, and/or amino acids

Week 1, Day 4

WHEN YOU WAKE UP
Tongue scraping and oil pulling (optional)

BEFORE BREAKFAST
Lemon water, 2 ounces of fresh wheatgrass, or 8 ounces of Mega Greens
     Drink (page 230)
Coffee enema
3 MAP capsules
30 minutes of yoga, Qigong, stretching, or walking
30 minutes of meditation, journaling, or prayer

BREAKFAST
Mocha Nut Milk Shake (page 232) or 1 or 2 Hard-Boiled Eggs (page 236),
     ½ avocado

MIDMORNING
2 ounces of wheatgrass

30 MINUTES BEFORE LUNCH
Cider Vinegar Drink (page 235)
3 MAP capsules

LUNCH
3 to 5 ounces of Dijon Dill Salmon (Recipes, page 272), 2 cups of baby
     greens, ½ cup of radishes, 1 tablespoon of MCT Essential Salad Dress-
     ing (page 249)

MIDAFTERNOON
8 ounces of Iced Green Tea (page 234)
15- to 30-minute walk, stretching, rebounding, or other exercise/activity

SNACK
8 Sprouted Nuts (page 279) or Toasted Nuts (page 280)

30 MINUTES BEFORE DINNER
1 cup of calming tea (e.g., chamomile)

DINNER
3 to 6 ounces of Versatile Meat Loaf (page 277), 2 cups of Baby Greens
    Side Salad (page 253), 1 tablespoon of MCT Essential Salad Dressing
    (page 249)

BEFORE BEDTIME
Fiber Drink (optional, page 235)
Epsom bath, sauna, body brushing, and/or another detoxification activity
Journaling, meditation, or prayer (if you didn't do in the morning)
For sleep: aromatherapy or Epsom salt bath, sleep audio, herbal supplements,
    melatonin, and/or amino acids

Week 1, Day 5

WHEN YOU WAKE UP
Tongue scraping and oil pulling (optional)

BEFORE BREAKFAST
Lemon water or Simply Greens Detox Beverage (page 228)
Coffee enema
4 MAP capsules
30 minutes of yoga, Qigong, stretching, or walking
30 minutes of meditation, journaling, or prayer

BREAKFAST
Whey or Plant Protein Powder Drink (page 233)

SNACK
8 ounces of Iced Green Tea (page 234) or Fresh Veggie Juice (page 229)
8 to 10 Sprouted Nuts (page 279) or Toasted Nuts (page 280)

30 MINUTES BEFORE LUNCH
2 ounces of wheatgrass, 8 ounces of Mega Greens Drink (page 230), or
    8 ounces of purified water (optional: add 1 teaspoon of cider vinegar)
4 MAP capsules

LUNCH
1 (3- to 5-ounce) Ground Chicken Patty (with Lettuce Wrap) (page 276),
    2 tablespoons of Fresh Guacamole (page 240), 2 tomato slices, 1 table-
    spoon of Spicy Burger Sauce (optional, page 239)

MIDAFTERNOON
2 ounces of wheatgrass or 8 ounces of Mega Greens Drink (page 230)
15- to 30-minute walk, stretch, rebounding, or other exercise/activity

SNACK
Whey or Plant Protein Powder Drink (page 233)

DINNER
Chinese Chicken Salad (page 255), 3 cups of romaine lettuce, 1 tablespoon
    of Cilantro Salad Dressing (page 250)

BEFORE BEDTIME
Fiber Drink (page 235)
Coffee enema, Epsom bath, sauna, and/or body brushing
Journaling, meditation, or prayer (if you didn't do in the morning)
For sleep: aromatherapy or Epsom salt bath, sleep audio, herbal supplements,
    melatonin, and/or amino acids

Week 1, Day 6

WHEN YOU WAKE UP
Tongue scraping and oil pulling (optional)

BEFORE BREAKFAST
Lemon water or Ginger Lemon Drink (page 229)
Coffee enema
4 MAP capsules
30 minutes of yoga, Qigong, stretching, or walking
30 minutes of meditation, journaling, or prayer

BREAKFAST
2 or 3 Poached Eggs (page 236), ½ avocado, 2 tomato slices

MIDMORNING
2 ounces of wheatgrass or 8 ounces of Ginger Lemon Drink (page 229)

BEFORE LUNCH
1 cup of green tea
4 MAP capsules

LUNCH
Chicken Vegetable Soup (page 263)

MIDAFTERNOON
Mega Greens Drink (page 230)
15- to 30-minute walk, stretch, rebounding, or other exercise/activity

SNACK
1 cup of green tea
10 Sprouted Nuts (page 279) or Toasted Nuts (page 280)

30 MINUTES BEFORE DINNER
Cider Vinegar Drink (optional, to aid in digestion) (page 235)

DINNER
1 (3- to 5-ounce Filet Mignon (page 272), 1 to 2 cups Steamed Cauliflower
    Delight (page 268)
1 cup of herbal tea

BEFORE BEDTIME
Fiber Drink (page 235)
Coffee enema, Epsom bath, sauna, and/or body brushing
Journaling, meditation, or prayer (if you didn't do in the morning)
For sleep: aromatherapy or Epsom salt bath, sleep audio, herbal supplements,
   melatonin, and/or amino acids

Week 1, Day 7

WHEN YOU WAKE UP
Tongue scraping and oil pulling (optional)

BEFORE BREAKFAST
Lemon water or Ginger Snap drink (page 227)
Coffee enema
5 MAP capsules
30 minutes of yoga, Qigong, stretching, or walking
30 minutes of meditation, journaling, or prayer

BREAKFAST
2 to 3 Hard-Boiled Eggs (page 236), 2 slices of Turkey Bacon (page 237),
   ½ avocado

SNACK
1 Raw Low-Carbohydrate Chocolate Square (page 282)

30 MINUTES BEFORE LUNCH
Cider Vinegar Drink (optional, page 235)
5 MAP capsules

LUNCH
1 (3–6-ounce) Ground Turkey Patty (with Lettuce Wrap) (page 276),
   1 tablespoon of Spicy Burger Sauce (page 239) or Mayonnaise (page
   238 or 239), ½ avocado

MIDAFTERNOON
Spicy Green drink (page 228)
15- to 30-minute walk, stretch, rebounding, or other exercise/activity

SNACK
1 cup of Savory Sipping Alkaline Broth (page 235)

30 MINUTES BEFORE DINNER
8 ounces of purified water
5 MAP capsules

DINNER
3.5 ounces of Ceviche Salad (page 257), ½ cup of chopped radish

BEFORE BEDTIME
Fiber Drink (page 235) or chamomile tea
Epsom bath, sauna, body brushing, and/or another detoxification activity
Journaling, meditation, or prayer (if you didn't do in the morning)
For sleep: aromatherapy or Epsom salt bath, sleep audio, herbal supplements,
      melatonin, and/or amino acids

Week 2, Day 8

WHEN YOU WAKE UP
Tongue scraping and oil pulling (optional)

BEFORE BREAKFAST
8 ounces of purified water or Savory Sipping Alkaline Broth (page 235)
Coffee enema
5 MAP capsules
30 minutes of yoga, Qigong, stretching, or walking
30 minutes of meditation, journaling, or prayer

BREAKFAST
Cinnamon Chia Pudding (page 282)

MIDMORNING
8 ounces of Spicy Green drink (page 228)

30 MINUTES BEFORE LUNCH
5 MAP capsules

LUNCH
Greek Salad with Chicken (page 254), 1 tablespoon of Citrus Delight Dress-
    ing (page 250)

MIDAFTERNOON
8 ounces of Iced Green Tea (page 234) or 8 ounces of Mega Greens Drink
    (page 230)
15- to 30-minute walk, stretching, rebounding, or other exercise/activity

30 MINUTES BEFORE DINNER
Ginger Snap drink (page 228)
5 MAP capsules

DINNER
3 to 5 ounces of Dijon Dill Salmon (page 272), 1 to 2 cups of steamed spin-
    ach, ½ avocado

BEFORE BEDTIME
Fiber Drink (page 235) or herbal tea
Epsom bath, sauna, body brushing, and/or another detoxification activity
Journaling, meditation, or prayer (if you didn't do in the morning)
For sleep: aromatherapy or Epsom salt bath, sleep audio, herbal supplements,
    melatonin, and/or amino acids

Week 2, Day 9

WHEN YOU WAKE UP
Tongue scraping and oil pulling (optional)

BEFORE BREAKFAST
Lemon water or Simply Greens Detox Beverage (page 228)
Coffee enema
6 MAP capsules
30 minutes of yoga, Qigong, stretching, or walking
30 minutes of meditation, journaling, or prayer

BREAKFAST
Whey or Plant Protein Powder Drink (page 233)

MIDMORNING
2 ounces of fresh wheatgrass or 8 ounces of Mega Greens Drink (page 230)

30 MINUTES BEFORE LUNCH
8 ounces of purified water
6 MAP capsules

LUNCH
3 to 5 ounces of Garlic Lemon Dijon Chicken (page 274), 1 to 2 cups of
    steamed broccoli

MIDAFTERNOON
Fresh Veggie Juice (page 229)
1 celery stick with almond butter
15- to 30-minute walk, stretching, rebounding, or other exercise/activity

30 MINUTES BEFORE DINNER
8 ounces of herbal or Iced Green Tea (page 234)
6 MAP capsules

BEFORE DINNER
Cider Vinegar Drink (optional, to aid in digestion) (page 235)

DINNER
3 to 5 ounces of Ceviche Salad (page 257), 2 cups of Baby Greens Side Salad
    (page 253), 1 tablespoon of MCT Essential Salad Dressing (page 249)

BEFORE BEDTIME
Fiber Drink (page 235) or herbal tea
Epsom bath, sauna, and/or body brushing
Journaling, meditation, or prayer (if you didn't do in the morning)
For sleep: aromatherapy or Epsom salt bath, sleep audio, herbal supplements,
　　　melatonin, and/or amino acids

Week 2, Day 10

WHEN YOU WAKE UP
Tongue scraping and oil pulling (optional)

BEFORE BREAKFAST
Lemon water or Savory Sipping Alkaline Broth (page 235)
6 MAP capsules
Coffee enema
30 minutes of yoga, Qigong, stretching or walking
30 minutes of meditation, journaling or prayer

BREAKFAST
Coco Loco Nut Shake (page 233)

MIDMORNING
2 ounces of fresh wheatgrass or 8 ounces of Mega Greens Drink (page 230)

30 MINUTES BEFORE LUNCH
Lemon/Limeade (page 234)
6 MAP capsules

LUNCH
3 to 6 ounces of Herb Almond Crusted Mahimahi (page 274), 1 to 2 cups of
　　　steamed asparagus, 1 tablespoon of MCT oil or organic butter

SNACK
8 Sprouted Nuts (page 279) or Toasted Nuts (page 280)

MIDAFTERNOON
8 ounces of purified water
6 MAP capsules
15- to 30-minute walk, stretch, rebounding, or other exercise/activity

DINNER
Note: For this meal, consider replacing your animal protein with MAP
capsules.

Nutty Greek Salad (page 254), 1 to 2 cups of Vegetable Medley Soup (page
    262), 1 tablespoon of MCT Essential Salad Dressing (page 249)
1 cup of chamomile tea

BEFORE BEDTIME
Fiber Drink (page 235)
Epsom bath, sauna, body brushing, and/or another detoxification activity
Journaling, meditation, or prayer (if you didn't do in the morning)
For sleep: aromatherapy or Epsom salt bath, sleep audio, herbal supplements,
    melatonin, and/or amino acids

Week 2, Day 11

WHEN YOU WAKE UP
Tongue scraping and oil pulling (optional)

BEFORE BREAKFAST
Lemon water or Savory Sipping Alkaline Broth (page 235)
Coffee enema
7 MAP capsules
30 minutes of yoga, Qigong, stretching, or walking
30 minutes of meditation, journaling, or prayer

BREAKFAST
Whey or Plant Protein Powder Drink (page 233)

SNACK
8 ounces of purified water or 2 ounces of fresh wheatgrass

30 MINUTES BEFORE LUNCH
8 ounces of Iced Green Tea (page 234)
7 MAP capsules

LUNCH
3 to 4 ounces of Seared Toasted Sesame Salmon Salad (page 258), 2 cups of
    Baby Greens Side Salad (page 253), 1 tablespoon Cilantro Salad Dress-
    ing (optional) (page 250)
1 cup of Savory Sipping Alkaline Broth (page 235)

MIDAFTERNOON
8 ounces of Iced Green Tea (page 234)
15- to 30-minute walk, stretch, rebounding, or other exercise/activity

SNACK
1 Raw Low-Carbohydrate Chocolate Square (page 282)

30 MINUTES BEFORE DINNER
1 cup of chamomile tea or Cider Vinegar Drink (optional) (page 235)
7 MAP capsules (to replace animal protein at dinner)

DINNER
Creamy Broccoli Soup (page 263), 2 cups of Greek Side Salad (page 254),
    ½ avocado, 1 tablespoon of MCT Essential Salad Dressing (page 249)

BEFORE BEDTIME
Fiber Drink (optional, page 235)
1 cup of Sleepytime tea (Celestial Seasonings)
Epsom bath, sauna, body brushing, and/or another detoxification activity
Journaling, meditation, or prayer (if you didn't do in the morning)
For sleep: aromatherapy or Epsom salt bath, sleep audio, herbal supplements,
    melatonin, and/or amino acids

Week 2, Day 12

WHEN YOU WAKE UP
Tongue scraping and oil pulling (optional)

BEFORE BREAKFAST
Lemon water
Coffee enema
7 MAP capsules
30 minutes of yoga, Qigong, stretching, or walking
30 minutes of meditation, journaling, or prayer

BREAKFAST
Whey or Plant Protein Powder Drink (page 233)

MIDMORNING
Mega Greens Drink (page 230)

30 MINUTES BEFORE LUNCH
8 ounces of purified water
7 MAP capsules

LUNCH
1 (3- to 6-ounce) Ground Chicken or Turkey Patty (with Lettuce Wrap)
    (page 276), Fresh Guacamole (page 240), 1 tablespoon of Mayonnaise
    (page 238 or 239) or gluten-free mustard

MIDAFTERNOON
2 ounces of fresh wheatgrass or 8 ounces of Mega Greens Drink (page 230)
15- to 30-minute walk, stretch, rebounding, or other exercise/activity

30 MINUTES BEFORE DINNER
7 MAP capsules (to replace protein at your evening meal)
1 cup of organic herbal tea

DINNER
1 to 2 cups of Curry Chicken Salad (page 256), 1 tablespoon of Cilantro
     Salad Dressing (page 250) or Creamy Curry Dip (page 244)

BEFORE BEDTIME
Fiber Drink (page 235)
1 cup of Sleepytime tea (Celestial Seasonings)
Epsom bath, sauna, body brushing, and/or another detoxification activity
Journaling, meditation, or prayer (if you didn't do in the morning)
For sleep: aromatherapy or Epsom salt bath, sleep audio, herbal supplements,
     melatonin, and/or amino acids

Week 2, Day 13

WHEN YOU WAKE UP
Tongue scraping and oil pulling (optional)

BEFORE BREAKFAST
8 ounces of lemon water
Coffee enema
8 MAP capsules
30 minutes of yoga, Qigong, stretching, or walking
30 minutes of meditation, journaling, or prayer

BREAKFAST
2 to 4 Poached Eggs (page 236), ½ avocado, 1 tablespoon of sriracha sauce
     (optional)

SNACK
1 to 2 ounces sliced turkey with Spicy Burger Sauce (page 239)

30 MINUTES BEFORE LUNCH
8 ounces of purified water
8 MAP capsules

LUNCH
Chicken Vegetable Soup (page 263)

MIDAFTERNOON
2 ounces of wheatgrass or 8 ounces of Mega Greens Drink (page 230)
15- to 30-minute walk, stretch, rebounding, or other exercise/activity

SNACK
1 cup of Savory Sipping Alkaline Broth (page 235)

30 MINUTES BEFORE DINNER
8 ounces of purified water with 1 teaspoon of cider vinegar
8 MAP capsules

DINNER
Optional: Replace animal protein at dinner with 8 MAP capsules (or an
amount commensurate with your body weight).
Nutty Greek Salad (page 254) or Curry Chicken Salad (page 256), 1 Steamed
     Artichoke (with Artichoke Dip) (page 267)
8 ounces of Iced Green Tea (page 234)

BEFORE BEDTIME
Epsom bath, sauna, and/or body brushing
Journaling, meditation, or prayer (if you didn't do in the morning)
Fiber Drink (page 235)
For sleep: aromatherapy or Epsom salt bath, sleep audio, herbal supplements,
     melatonin, and/or amino acids

Week 2, Day 14

WHEN YOU WAKE UP
Tongue scraping and oil pulling (optional)

BEFORE BREAKFAST
Lemon water or Ginger Lemon Drink (page 229)
Coffee enema

8 MAP capsules
30 minutes of yoga, Qigong, stretching, or walking
30 minutes of meditation, journaling, or prayer

BREAKFAST
Whey or Plant Protein Powder Drink (page 233)

MIDMORNING
2 ounces of wheatgrass or 8 ounces of Mega Greens Drink (page 230)

30 MINUTES BEFORE LUNCH
8 ounces of purified water or green tea
8 MAP capsules

LUNCH
3 to 6 ounces of Versatile Meat Loaf (page 277), Creamy Cauliflower Soup
    (page 263)

MIDAFTERNOON
15- to 30-minute walk, stretch, rebounding, or other exercise/activity
2 ounces of wheatgrass or 8 ounces Ginger Snap drink (page 228)

30 MINUTES BEFORE DINNER
Cider Vinegar Drink (page 235)
8 MAP capsules (to replace animal protein at evening meal)

DINNER
Zucchini Noodles (page 271) with Parsley Pesto (page 242), Greek Side Salad
    (page 254)

BEFORE BEDTIME
Fiber Drink (page 235)
1 cup of Sleepytime tea (Celestial Seasonings)
Epsom bath, sauna, body brushing, and/or another detoxification activity
Journaling, meditation, or prayer (if you didn't do in the morning)
For sleep: aromatherapy or Epsom salt bath, sleep audio, herbal supplements,
    melatonin, and/or amino acids

You can use this chart to help track your daily progress: photocopy it and paste it into your journal or re-create it on your computer. It's a great go-to for keeping track of your healing journey.

14-DAY PLAN DAILY TRACKER

Supplements:	Dosage:

DETOXIFICATION

Rebounding (1–3 times/day):	
Oil pulling or tongue brushing (First thing in the morning before eating, drinking, or brushing):	
Bowel movements (Note any changes or unusual bowel movements.):	
Coffee enema (1x/day):	
Rebounding (1–3 times/day):	
Oil pulling or tongue brushing (First thing in the morning before eating, drinking, or brushing):	
Bowel movements (Note any changes or unusual bowel movements.):	
Coffee enema (1x/day):	

EXERCISE

Walking or other exercise (minimum 30 minutes/day):	
Sunshine (15 minutes/day):	

pH Reading:

Weight:

Water Intake:

Juice Intake:

Breakfast:

Lunch:

Dinner:

Snacks:

Sleep:	Bedtime:	Wake time:	# Times wakeup:	Hours slept:

Notes:

"You become what you think about most of the time."

A Word About pH and the Ketogenic Diet

> **NOTE:** The ketogenic diet is generally thought to be unsafe for people with diabetes. It may also be contraindicated in some other health conditions or situations. When done properly, it can have powerful anticancer effects, but whether it is appropriate for you will depend upon your unique constitution and situation, and it is therefore best to consult with your doctor before starting it.

Whenever you follow a high-fat, moderate protein, and low-carbohydrate diet, your body will start to produce ketones for energy, rather than glucose. Ketones are water-soluble by-products created when your body breaks down fatty acids for energy. It is normal and good for your body to produce ketones while you are on a ketogenic food plan, but if the amount of ketones in your body increases too much (which can happen when you aren't consuming enough carbohydrates), then your blood pH can become too acidic. This can occasionally lead to a serious problem called ketoacidosis (I discuss symptoms of ketoacidosis on page 199). Again, people with certain types of cancer or health conditions may be more susceptible to ketoacidosis, so I highly recommend that you consult with your doctor before you begin this diet.

You'll also want to periodically monitor and balance your pH while on the ketogenic diet by measuring your body's daily production of ketones. You can do this with a blood ketone meter, which you can purchase at many retail box stores, your local pharmacy, or online.

You can also make sure that your pH is balanced by consuming ample amounts of minerals, especially magnesium, potassium, calcium, and trace minerals. Minerals neutralize acids that are produced during the initial stages of the diet. Additionally, it's a good idea to drink alkalinizing water and consume alkalinizing foods, such as Mega Greens, as green drinks balance your body's pH and help prevent electrolyte imbalances. I also recommend taking bile salts, no matter what diet you are on, but especially while doing the ketogenic diet. Bile salts help your body digest fats. If you have had your gallbladder removed, taking bile salts is absolutely essential. But again, consult your doctor before making a change to your treatment regimen.

How to Measure Your Body's Production of Ketones

Urine sticks, which are a popular method for measuring the amount of ketones your body produces, tend to only work well during the first few weeks that you are in ketosis and don't provide real-time results. That means if you test yourself at two p.m., you will get a reading that reflects what your ketone levels were at noon, not two p.m. For better results, use a blood ketone meter, such as Abbott's Precision Xtra meter, which you can purchase online, at Walmart, or at your local pharmacy. These meters aren't too expensive, they are easy to use, and they provide accurate, real-time results.

When testing, you want the ketone reading to be within a range of 2 to 8. If the value is lower than 2, that means you aren't using fat for energy (and are instead burning glucose) and need to consume fewer carbohydrate-containing foods. If it is higher than 8, then you are producing too many ketones and putting your body at risk for ketoacidosis, and you'll want to either consume more carbohydrate-containing foods or switch to a different food plan.

Symptoms of ketoacidosis include:

- Constantly feeling tired
- Dry and flushed skin
- Nausea, vomiting, or abdominal pain
- Difficulty breathing
- Fruity odor on the breath
- Difficulty focusing, brain fog, or confusion

If you experience any of these symptoms, consult your doctor. It is normal to experience some tiredness, irritability, or brain fog during the first week or two that you are on a ketogenic diet, but if your symptoms persist long term or are serious, and include such symptoms as nausea or trouble breathing, then this means you are either producing too many ketones or that the diet isn't suitable for you. To learn more about the ketogenic diet, you may also want to consult one of the many good books on the topic, such as *Keto Clarity: Your Definitive Guide to the Benefits of a Low-Carb, High-Fat Diet.*

Ketogenic Diet Portion Guidelines

The following are approximate food portion guidelines that we recommend if you are on a ketogenic food plan. These are similar to the portions recommended in the 14-day plan. The actual portion size you need will depend upon many factors, including your current health condition and your weight. As I mentioned earlier, people require different carbohydrate amounts to go into ketosis; anywhere from 0 to 50 grams daily, although the average is somewhere between 15 and 25 grams, so aiming for a diet that is somewhere within this range is recommended. The amount of carbohydrates that you will be able to consume also depends on whether you are a fast or slow oxidizer; that is, whether you metabolize food quickly or slowly.

Similarly, the amount of protein and fat you'll want to consume on a ketogenic diet depends on your unique constitution. Generally, you don't need to watch your fat consumption as much while on this type of food plan, but it is possible to eat too much protein, so the following food intake guidelines will help you determine exactly how much of each type of food to consume daily. Basically, your daily intake of protein, carbohydrates, and good fats should fall within the following ranges:

Protein: 60–75 grams daily = 15–20% of your total daily intake = 300 calories
Carbohydrates: 15–25 grams daily = 3–5% of your daily food intake = 750 calories
Fats: 112–125 grams daily = 75% of your daily food intake = 1,125 calories

You generally don't need to count calories on a ketogenic food plan, but if you wish to do so, you can use the following guidelines as a reference to determine your personal calorie prescription:

1 gram of fat = 9 calories
1 gram of MCT oil = 10 calories
1 gram of protein = 4 calories
1 gram of carbohydrates = 4 calories

How to Calculate Your Personal Protein Prescription

If you are healthy and don't have any medical reason to restrict protein in your diet, you should aim to eat about one-third (0.33) to one-half (0.50) gram of protein per day, per pound of body weight. Or convert your weight into kilograms, which you can do by dividing your weight by 2.2, and that will tell you about how many grams of protein you need on a daily basis. If you are heading into surgery or recovering from surgery, you may need more protein—as much as 0.65 to 0.80 grams of protein per pound of body weight.

The following is the formula for calculating your personal protein prescription:

__ pounds × 0.33 grams/pound = __ grams (calculate from your ideal weight)
Or __ pounds × 0.50 grams/pound = __ grams (calculate from your ideal weight)

Simply insert your weight into the first blank, and multiply by 0.33 or by 0.50 (if you need more protein) to get your total daily protein intake, in grams.

So, for instance, if you weighed 170 pounds and wanted to consume smaller amounts of protein, you would multiply your weight by 0.33 to get your daily intake of protein, which would be 56.1 grams. Then, you would divide that by three to get your ideal protein intake per meal, which in this case would be 18.7. If you needed more protein, you would multiply 170 by 0.50, to get 85 grams of protein daily. You would then divide that by 3 to calculate your protein intake per meal, which in this instance would be 28.3. If you are malnourished, underweight, or recovering from surgery, you would multiply your weight by 0.65 to 0.80 to get your daily intake. For a 170-pound person, this would amount to 110.5 to 136 grams of protein daily.

As a final note, your body begins to use fat for fuel about 3 hours after your last meal. So, if possible, spread your meals apart by four to five hours. This will encourage your body to use fats for fuel and ketosis, rather than glucose, for its energy production needs.

Low-Carb/Ketogenic Anticancer Foods

The following foods are healthy for anyone on a ketogenic diet, as well as for most anyone who is following a relatively low-carbohydrate or anticancer diet that may or may not be ketogenic.

Grass-Fed Organic Meat, Seafood, and Poultry

Most people will need anywhere from 15 to 30 grams of animal protein per meal, based on their personal protein prescription calculation. Again, the exact amount you'll need depends on your weight, constitution, and other factors, as discussed on page 200. The following are acceptable sources of animal protein. A 4-ounce serving of most of the following contains about 25–30 grams of protein. Most of the meals in the 14-day plan include 3.5 to 4 ounces of protein. If you are following a ketogenic diet and want to calculate the exact number of grams of protein, fat, and carbohydrate in your foods, there are many online food counters that can help you do this, as the portions provided in the 14-day plan are simply an approximation of what an average person might need. Some good ones include My Fitness Pal: www.myfitnesspal.com and My Food Diary: www.myfooddiary.com. See the Resources for more information.

HEALTHY PROTEIN FOOD SOURCES

Beef, Poultry, Lamb, and Game

Beef (grass-fed)	Turkey, ground
Chicken breast, skinless	Turkey bacon, 4 strips
Chicken breast, deli	Turkey/chicken sausage, 4 links
Lamb	Wild game meat (bison,
Turkey breast, skinless	venison, elk, etc.)
Turkey breast, deli-style	

Fish and Seafood

Bass (freshwater)	Mackerel*
Bass (sea)	Salmon*
Bluefish	Sardine*
Calamari	Snapper
Catfish	Swordfish
Cod	Shrimp
Clams	Trout
Crabmeat	Tuna (Albacore steak)
Haddock	Tuna (Albacore canned in
Halibut	water), 1 ounce
Lobster	

(* = rich in EPA)

Note: Tuna has been found to have higher levels of mercury than some other types of fish, so consuming it only occasionally is recommended, unless you buy from a reputable company, such as Vital Choice Seafood, which offers low-mercury tuna. See the Resources for more information.

Eggs

Organic egg, 1 (if you aren't allergic to eggs)
Egg whites, 2 (if you aren't allergic to eggs)

Vegetarian Protein-Based Foods

Note: The following represent an average serving size on a low-carb or ketogenic diet.

Vegan raw seed cheese: 2 ounces = 10 grams of protein
Chia seeds: 2 tablespoons = 5 grams of protein
Hemp seeds: 3 tablespoons = 11 grams of protein
Plant-based protein powder (usually 14–21 grams of protein per scoop; see Resources for product recommendations)
MAP: 6 to 10 capsules (can replace a serving of animal protein)

Low-Carbohydrate Vegetables

All of the following vegetables are delicious, nutritious options for the ketogenic or any other anticancer, low-carb food plan. If you are on a ketogenic food plan, choose one of the following vegetables to accompany each meal, along with a simple salad (see the Recipes section), or consult your physician or nutritionist for guidance.

Carbohydrates should consist of 3 to 5 percent of your total calories if you want to remain in ketosis. Two cups of nonstarchy vegetables contains 10 to 25 calories. If you aren't following a ketogenic food plan, you can consume higher amounts of most of the following foods. For each of these, we provide a recommended serving size to stay in ketosis, but you will want to adjust the serving size according to your needs.

COOKED VEGETABLES (AND RECOMMENDED SERVING SIZES)

Artichoke, 1 medium-size	Brussels sprouts, 1½ cups
Artichoke hearts, 1½ cups	Cabbage, 1 cup
Asparagus (12 spears), 1 cup	Carrot, 1 whole
Beans (green or wax), 1 cup	Cauliflower, 1½ cups
Bok choy, 2 cups	Collard greens, 1 cup
Broccoli, 2 cups	Eggplant, 1½ cups

Kale, 2 cups	Swiss chard, 1 cup
Leeks, 1 cup	Turnip, mashed, 1½ cups
Mushrooms (portobello), 1 cup	Turnip greens, 2 cups
Onion, chopped, ½ cup	Yellow squash, 1 cup
Okra, sliced, 1 cup	Zucchini, 2 cups
Spinach, 2 cups	

RAW VEGETABLES (AND RECOMMENDED SERVING SIZES)

Alfalfa sprouts, 2 cups	Onion, chopped, ½ cup
Bamboo shoots, 2 cups	Radishes, sliced, 2 cups
Bean sprouts, 2 cups	Salsa, ½ cup
Cabbage, shredded, 2 cups	Sea vegetables: dulse (2 table-
Cauliflower pieces, 2 cups	spoons), nori (3 sheets),
Celery, sliced, 2 cups	wakame (¾ cup),
Cucumber, sliced, 2 cups	kelp (2 tablespoons)
Endive, chopped, 2 cups	Snow peas, 1½ cups
Escarole, chopped, 2 cups	Spinach, 3 cups
Green or red peppers, 1½ cups	Tomato, 1 medium-size
Lettuce, baby greens, 2 cups	Tomatoes, cherry, 3
Lettuce, romaine, chopped, 2 cups	Water chestnuts, ⅓ cup

Healthy Fats

The following fatty foods are all great to eat on any low-carb anticancer or ketogenic diet. I would recommend consuming fat with every meal, especially coconut or MCT oil, which are metabolically active fats that help support ketosis. Recommended serving sizes are also included here.

Fat digestion is greatly enhanced when the fats are eaten with cultured vegetables, daikon, leafy green salads, cider vinegar, and lemon juice. Avoid unhealthy saturated and hydrogenated fats, and limit your intake of mono-saturated fats. One tablespoon of most oils contains about 100 calories, or 15 grams of fat; a tablespoon of most nut butters contains about 7 grams of fat. If you want to make sure to keep your carbohydrate intake low, you'll want to emphasize oils over nut butters in your diet, since nut butters also contain carbohydrates, which can increase your daily intake of carbs too much.

HEALTHY FATS (AND RECOMMENDED SERVING SIZES)

Almond or other nut butter,
    2 tablespoons

Almonds, 5

Avocado, ½ avocado or
    3 tablespoons

Coconut oil, 1 tablespoon

Guacamole, 2 tablespoons

Macadamia nuts, 4

Malaysian palm oil, 1 tablespoon

MCT oil, 1 tablespoon

Olives, 6

Olive oil, 1 tablespoon

Organic butter, 1 tablespoon

Pumpkin seed oil, 1 tablespoon

Slivered almonds, 1 teaspoon

Tahini, 1 tablespoon

Walnuts, chopped, 1 tablespoon

MODERATELY HEALTHY FATS (AND RECOMMENDED SERVING SIZES)

Ghee (clarified butter), 1 teaspoon

Organic mayonnaise, 1 tablespoon

Sesame oil, 1 teaspoon

A Note About Copper-Containing Foods

Copper is an essential mineral your body uses to make bone and connective tissue, as well as code specific enzymes. Your body needs this mineral in trace amounts, so you generally won't need to supplement for deficiencies unless your physician advises you to do so. However, in excess, copper can be poisonous, and may encourage cancer growth and cause other problems in people that have compromised immune function. To avoid the problems associated with copper toxicity, you may not want to consume large amounts of the following foods, all of which contain copper. The amount of copper in these foods is listed from greatest to least. You can also have your physician test your copper levels through a simple blood test before adding these foods to your diet on a regular basis.

Beef liver: 12 mg per 3 ounces

Oysters, lobster, crab, and octopus: 5.71 mg copper per 3 ounces, or
    about 6 oysters

Sesame seeds: 5.88 mg per cup, or 1.14 mg per ounce

Cashews: 3.4 mg per cup, or 0.62 mg per ounce. All nuts have some
    copper. Almonds, pecans, and pistachios have the lowest amounts.

Kale: 1.5 mg per cup

Mushrooms: 0.9 mg per cup, or about 4 mushrooms

Chickpeas, cooked: 0.58 mg per cup. All beans have some copper, with
white beans having the lowest amount.

Avocado: 0.44 mg per cup

Goat cheese: 0.21 mg per ounce

Unfiltered tap water

Essential Anticancer "Superfoods" and Their Benefits

In addition to the foods listed in this chapter, you'll want to include ample amounts of some or all of the following key anticancer foods and nutrients in your daily food plan.

Turmeric and curry. These are powerful anti-inflammatory spices that stimulate cancer cell death and inhibit tumor blood vessel growth.

Ginger has anti-inflammatory properties and antioxidant effects that are greater than those that are found in vitamin E. It can help reduce tumor blood vessel growth, and symptoms of nausea and vomiting that may be caused by conventional cancer treatments.

Cruciferous vegetables, such as cabbage, Brussels sprouts, bok choy, Chinese cabbage, broccoli, and cauliflower, contain sulforaphane and indole-3 carbinols (I3Cs), which are powerful anticancer molecules. Avoid boiling these vegetables, as boiling destroys the sulforaphane and I3Cs.

Garlic, onions, leeks, shallots, and chives. These all contain sulfur compounds that reduce the carcinogenic effects of nitrosamines and other compounds that are created when meat is grilled or overcooked. They also promote cancer cell death in many types of cancer. Garlic, an antibacterial, is one of the most powerful anticancer foods you can eat.

Carrots, celery, cucumber, grapefruit, and parsley all have an antioxidant effect on the body.

Tomatoes also have an antioxidative effect upon the body. The lycopene in tomatoes has been linked to increased survival times in men with prostate cancer.

Mushrooms. Shiitake, maitake, cremini, portobello, oyster, and thistle oyster mushrooms all contain polysaccharides and lentinan that stimulate the reproduction and activity of immune cells.

Herbs and spices, such as rosemary, thyme, oregano, basil, parsley, and mint, all promote cancer cell death. They also may help reduce the spread of cancer by blocking enzymes that the cancer needs to invade neighboring tissues. Cilantro helps bind with heavy metals so that the body can more easily eliminate them.

Seaweed. Several varieties of seaweed, also known as sea vegetables, such as kombu and wakame, contain molecules that are linked to slowed cancer growth, especially in breast, prostate, skin, and colon cancers. Nori is a sea vegetable that contains long-chain omega-3 fatty acids, and is the most effective of the seaweeds for combating inflammation.

Omega-3 essential fatty acids (EFAs). Long-chain omega-3 EFAs found in fatty fish (or high-quality purified fish oil supplements) reduce inflammation and the spread of cancer cells.

Selenium-rich foods, such as Brazil nuts, tuna, and sunflower seeds, can help stimulate the production of natural killer (NK) and other immune cells, as well as the body's antioxidant mechanisms.

Vitamin D. Vitamin D can help reduce cancer risk. Getting just twenty minutes of noonday sun exposure over your entire body can provide you with 8,000 to 10,000 IUs of vitamin D (note, though, that extended exposure beyond twenty minutes, without sun protection, can pose potential risks). Alternatively, take a vitamin D_3 supplement.

Probiotics. The intestines ordinarily contain beneficial or "friendly" bacteria, which improve digestion and facilitate regular bowel movements. Among the most common of these are *Lactobacillus acidophilus* and *Lactobacillus bifidus*. Studies suggest these probiotics may inhibit the growth of colon cancer cells.

Berries. Strawberries, raspberries, blueberries, blackberries, and cranberries contain ellagic acid and are rich in polyphenols. These properties may help eliminate carcinogenic substances and inhibit tumor blood vessel growth. Anthocyanidins and proanthocyanidins, flavonoids that are found in berries, also may promote cancer cell death.

Citrus fruit. Oranges, tangerines, lemons, and grapefruit contain anti-inflammatory flavonoids. They also stimulate the liver to more effectively help detoxify carcinogenic substances.

Pomegranate. This fruit contains anti-inflammatory and antioxidant properties, and studies suggest it may reduce the recurrence of prostate and other types of cancer.

Red wine. This drink contains polyphenols, including resveratrol, which may help slow the spread of cancer cells. Pinot noir is particularly rich in resveratrol. However, it's best to not drink more than one glass of wine daily because too much may actually increase cancer incidence. Wine is also generally contraindicated on the ketogenic diet, so you'll want to avoid it if you are on this, or another very low-carb diet. Consult your doctor before consuming red wine.

Dark organic chocolate. Chocolate that is comprised of more than 70% cocoa contains high amounts of antioxidants, proanthocyanidins, and polyphenols. In fact, a single square of chocolate can contain twice as much of these as a glass of red wine or almost as much as a cup of green tea. These molecules may help slow the growth of cancer cells and inhibit angiogenesis. Avoid mixing dairy products with dark chocolate, as this cancels out the beneficial effects of the chocolate. Consume chocolate sparingly as an occasional treat, and no more than one or two squares at a time.

JUANITA'S Story

I have found that establishing a morning, afternoon, and evening routine has been essential for helping me remember to complete all aspects of my treatment regimen. I schedule my activities and make a list of all the things that I need to do, which helps me save my "brain power" for the other important things that I need to think about during the day. So, for instance, my morning "to-do" list might include such things as taking my vitamins, making a wheatgrass drink, or jumping on a trampoline for ten minutes. Then I have a different schedule for the afternoons and evenings.

I keep the schedule containing my to-do list inside a plastic sheet protector and use an Expo marker to place a check mark after every activity that I complete during the day. At the end of the day, I review the list to see what I have remembered or forgotten to do, so that the things that I forgot to do then become an important part of my agenda for the next day. So, for instance, if I forget to do a detox bath or a coffee enema one day, the list helps me remember to do those things the next day and to evaluate what pieces of my healing puzzle that I need to focus more on.

Having a routine also helps me adjust my treatments according to my schedule because I have found that different treatments work in different places and situations, and some things take more time and preparation than others. For instance, if I'm at home all day, I might do a coffee enema. If I am away from home all day, I'll skip the enema and do that treatment the following day.

Following a complete cancer regimen can be time consuming, and I've had to give up some of my other daily activities so that I have more time to focus on my health, but I believe that it is well worth it because if you only do half of the program, you will only get half of the results.

CHAPTER 13

The 7-Day Juicing Detoxification Program

IN THIS CHAPTER, YOU WILL FIND . . .

- A 7-day juicing detoxification plan that will help you to eliminate environmental toxins and metabolic waste from your body
- Exercise suggestions to improve the detoxification process

Juicing and juice fasting are used in many cultures for their potential medicinal purposes, especially to cleanse the body of unwanted waste and boost immunity. Today, juicing has become a mainstream practice in the United States, and more and more people are joining the juicing revolution to help beat cancer or simply maintain their health.

I highly recommend adding juicing to your daily wellness regimen for several reasons. First, juicing can give you energy and provide instantaneous, noticeable positive results in your mood and sense of well-being, which can be a powerful motivational factor that spurs you on to meet your health goals. You'll likely notice juicing increases your energy, clears up your brain fog, restores your digestion, and/or reduces other symptoms. It also cleanses your cells and gives your organs a rest from having to digest and metabolize solid food. Finally, it boosts your immune system and conserves your body's energy to help fight or ward off disease.

In this chapter I will be sharing with you a 7-day juicing and exercise program that has the potential to help you to detoxify and strengthen your body. Although you will not be eating any solid foods on this program, you will still be getting all of the nutrients you need during the juice fast, as juices retain 95 percent of all of the nutrients found in whole fruits and vegetables. You are also not likely to feel hungry during the program because you will be consuming some plant-based protein powders that will give you strength and help to keep your blood sugar balanced.

Although this program is seven days long, you can also shorten it to fit your schedule and needs. For instance, you could do a 3-day plan and follow Days 1 to 3 of the plan, or do a 5-day plan and follow Days 1 to 5. So, if you can't do a full seven days, that's okay! Just pat yourself on the back for whatever you are able to do, and if you are able to juice for a full seven days, that's great! While this program focuses on juicing and exercise, for greater impact and benefit, you can also add to it any of the other do-it-yourself detoxification strategies described in Chapter 5, such as a sauna, Epsom salt baths, or body brushing.

As a final note, if you are too tired or don't have the energy or time to make all of the juices described in this chapter, you can purchase ready-made vegetable juices at your local health food store, grocery store, or juice bar (see the guidelines on how to choose healthy juices in Chapter 4, page 66). You will still reap most of the benefits of this fast by doing it this way. Juice bars are becoming increasingly common across the United States, and some nationwide companies, such as Jamba Juice, now make several cold-pressed green veggie juices that are healthy and delicious. Many juice companies also offer national shipping, so no matter where you are, you can even purchase fresh juices for delivery to your home!

Prep and Side Effects

If you have been following the 14-day plan, by now your body will have rid itself of some toxins as a result of eating purely healthy foods, and thus will be better prepared to take on the 7-day program. In fact, I highly recommend completing the 14-day plan before starting this program, as it will minimize any undesirable detoxification symptoms you may experience from juicing, and which are caused by your body's dumping a large amount of toxins all at once. They can include such things as feeling spacey, irritable, lightheaded, or hungry, especially after the first two days on the juicing program. If you happen to experience these symptoms anyway, you can add more protein powder to any of the following recipes, provided that the protein you use is plant-based. You may also want to eat just vegetables for a couple of days before and after the fast, as this will help to prepare your body for it.

If you feel that you need more sustenance on this plan, you can also substitute the blended juice recipes mentioned in the Recipes section at the end of this book for any of the juices mentioned here. The juices in the Recipes section contain fiber, and as such, may feel a bit heavier in your stomach than some of the juices listed here. See pages 227–231 of the Recipes section for more information.

Finally, if you are weak or have lost a lot of weight as a result of conventional cancer treatments, or have another medical condition that might preclude fasting, consult your doctor before doing this program to make sure it is safe and appropriate for you. He or she might recommend that you try out a shorter fast lasting one to two days instead, or simply wait until you are stronger or more rehabilitated.

Above all, be sure to ask your doctor before trying this fast.

Exercise and Juicing

I also recommend that, as part of the 7-day program, you do some moderate exercise daily, which will further help your body to eliminate toxins. In particular, I recommend rebounding, which is a great, low-impact exercise that can help stimulate your lymphatic system and help your body to "take out the garbage" (toxins) and "bring in the groceries" (nutrients from the juices). You can purchase a rebounder, or mini-trampoline, at most sporting goods stores.

Rebounders are great because you can do a wide variety of exercises on them, from light ankle bounces to single leg jumps, squat jumps or side lunges. You can even do twists and jumping jacks. You can get creative and even break a sweat if you like. Rebounding is an amazing way to get into shape, and it is the only exercise that uses every single muscle in the body. I highly recommend rebounding outside in the sun as a way to get your daily dose of vitamin D and stimulate your body's production of mood-enhancing serotonin.

Alternatively, you can take a walk daily, which will also facilitate toxin removal, by stimulating your circulation and lymphatic system, and by oxygenating your tissues, especially if you walk up and down a varied terrain. You don't need to do strenuous exercise as part of the 7-day program; just do something active for thirty minutes or longer every day. But ideally, you want it to be an activity that will stimulate your lymphatic system and cause you to sweat a little.

Daily Journaling

As part of the 7-day detox program, you'll also want to keep a daily journal about your experience so you can evaluate how you felt throughout the process. The following are some questions to ponder and write about in your journal during and after the program, which will help you get the most out of your detoxification program and refine it for the future.

1. How did you feel each day of the program?
2. Which juices did you like the most?
3. Were you able to incorporate at least thirty minutes of exercise into your daily routine, and if so, which exercises did you do?
4. How did these exercises make you feel?
5. How do you feel now, after having finished the 7-day program?
6. On a scale of 1 to 10, rate the overall change in your energy level.
7. During the program, did you drink only juice, or did you add protein powder or other foods to the program?
8. Were you hungry on any of the days?
9. How was your mental clarity before, during, and after the process?
10. What did you discover about yourself as a result of the 7-day program?

Postfasting Considerations

As I mentioned earlier in this chapter, once you finish the fast, it is a good idea to reintroduce solid foods to your body slowly, as your body will have become accustomed to consuming only liquids. This process should only take a couple of days. Start with some fruits and veggies, and on the third day, add some light protein. You might try a baby greens, arugula, or kale side salad, or some cooked veggies, such as fennel with turmeric, steamed dilled carrots, roasted zucchini and eggplant, steamed cauliflower, or vegetable soup during the first two days. See the Recipes section for information on how to prepare these dishes. On the third day, you might add in a Greek salad, some eggs or turkey bacon, or a hearty chicken vegetable or beef soup. After that, you can go back to your full meal plan, which might include heavier meals with larger amounts of protein.

During this time, I encourage you to reflect upon how you feel. Look over the journal that you maintained, and rate your overall experience during the program. Then give yourself a big high five for all that you learned about yourself, your body, and your mind, and for the positive changes that you made to your health!

Juicing Tools and Ingredients

To make the following juices, you will need:

- A juicer (a centrifugal or slow-masticating cold-press juicer is best)
- A quality blender or Vitamix
- Vegetable scrubber
- Grape seed extract (GSE) for rinsing all your produce. GSE cleanses and eliminates parasites on produce.
- Glass containers to store the washed vegetables
- Mason jars to store the juice
- Organic produce
- Psyllium husks. These are an excellent fiber that will aid in eliminating toxins. Once inside the intestines, the psyllium traps and removes toxins that might otherwise accumulate and back up into your body, and cause such symptoms as headaches, loss of energy, and fatigue. As a bulking agent, psyllium also creates a sense of fullness. You can take this fiber several times daily in water or add it to your freshly prepared juices. The fiber bulks up quickly, so drink it immediately after mixing it in your beverages; otherwise, you may have to eat your drink with a spoon!
- Protein powder from a vegetarian source. Plant-based protein provides amino acids to your body and supports detoxification.
- A high-quality probiotic, to aid in repopulating the gut with beneficial bacteria and destroying pathogens, such as *Candida*.
- Organic spirulina powder. This tiny aquatic plant, which is 60 percent protein, is bursting with essential vitamins and phytonutrients, such as the antioxidant beta-carotene and the essential fatty

acid GLA. It also contains a high amount of chlorophyll to support alkalinity.

- Stevia (optional, to sweeten the juices)

Tips for Top Juices and Basic Juice Instructions

- Rinse all your produce with grape seed extract (GSE). GSE cleanses and eliminates parasites on produce. Add 20 drops to a large bowl of water.
- For all the following recipes, simply place the washed vegetables and/or fruits, one at a time, in a juicer and turn on the juicer. Process until you get the desired amount of juice for each vegetable or fruit.
- You can prepare all the juices for the day each morning and store them in mason jars in the refrigerator for later use, or prepare them fresh throughout the day. I recommend making 32 to 36 ounces of each juice and then mixing them together as needed to make the appropriate recipes. So, for example, if on one day your total carrot juice intake is 32 ounces, or is 36 ounces of cucumber, you would juice the total quantity from each one of these vegetables and store them separately in mason jars, and then when it comes time to make a recipe that combines, you will mix the different varieties of juices together.
- If you wish to add avocado or protein powder to any of the recipes, simply mix the juice, along with the avocado or protein powder, in a blender or Vitamix.
- The juices are best consumed fresh—if not immediately then the day they are made.
- Start each day with warm lemon water (juice of ½ lemon in 8 ounces of water) or hot mint tea.

Recipes for the 7-Day Plan

Lemon Ginger Turmeric Juice

1 large pink grapefruit
1 orange
Juice of 1 lemon
1 cup purified water

1 (⅓-inch-long) piece fresh turmeric
1 (⅓-inch-long) piece fresh ginger
Stevia, to taste (optional)

Super-Duper Juice

½ large cucumber
1 cup fresh parsley
6 Swiss chard leaves
4 celery stalks
4 cups spinach
8 large kale leaves
3 medium-size carrots

Vital Greens Juice

4 medium-size carrots
8 cups spinach
1 tablespoon freshly squeezed lemon juice
1 medium-size beet
1 apple
(Optional: Add ½ avocado or plant-based protein powder, such as hemp, to this recipe after you've juiced the produce.)

Mineral Refresh Juice

7 cups spinach
½ large cucumber
1 apple
4 celery stalks
1 cup fresh parsley

The Stabilizer Juice

3 carrots
10 romaine or other lettuce leaves
8 string beans (1 ounce)
½ cucumber
3 celery stalks

Citrus Magic

1 large pink grapefruit
1 orange
Juice of 1 lemon
Handful of fresh mint
1 (⅓-inch) piece fresh ginger
4 to 6 ounces purified water
Stevia, to taste (optional)

Super Ruby Greens

1 medium-size beet
4 medium-size carrots
½ cabbage head
4 celery stalks
1 garlic clove
1 cup fresh cilantro

The Emerald

6 cups spinach
¾ large cucumber
1 apple
4 celery stalks
1 cup fresh parsley or cilantro (optional)

The following are a couple of additional juices you can use in place of any of those just listed, for greater variety. As part of the 7-day juice fast, you may also add broth to your recipes (see Savory Sipping Alkaline Broth, page 235).

Meta Boost

This juice blend has a diuretic effect and may help your body flush out any unwanted fat deposits and toxins. It may also help to speed up your metabolism.

4 carrots
6 cups spinach

4 cups cabbage
Juice of ½ lemon
1 large kale leaf
½ medium-size cucumber

Clarity Blend

This juice is high in potassium. Potassium can help your body maintain a healthy nervous system and optimal brain function. There are high amount of vitamins, minerals, and antioxidants in this juice, including vitamins A, B_9, C, D, and K; iron, calcium, CoQ10, and sulforaphane, to support detoxification.

1 cup broccoli, with stalks
4 carrots
4 cups spinach
1 apple
½ medium-size cucumber

7-Day Plan Menus

DAY 1

7 a.m. (or first thing in the morning): Warm lemon water or hot mint tea
8 a.m.: Lemon Ginger Turmeric Juice
11 a.m.: Super-Duper Juice
2 p.m.: Vital Greens Juice
5 p.m.: Mineral Refresh
8 p.m.: The Stabilizer Juice
9 p.m.: Mint, Sleepytime (Celestial Seasonings), or chamomile tea

DAY 2

7 a.m.: Warm lemon water or hot mint tea
8 a.m.: Citrus Magic
11 a.m.: Super Ruby Greens
2 p.m.: The Emerald
5 p.m.: Super Ruby Greens

8 p.m.: Lemon Ginger Turmeric Juice

9 p.m.: Mint, Sleepytime, or chamomile tea

DAY 3

7 a.m.: Warm lemon water or hot mint tea

8 a.m.: Lemon Ginger Turmeric Juice

11 a.m.: Super-Duper Juice

2 p.m.: Vital Greens

5 p.m.: Lemon Ginger Turmeric Juice

8 p.m.: The Stabilizer

9 p.m.: Mint, Sleepytime, or chamomile tea

DAY 4

7 a.m.: Warm lemon water or hot mint tea

8 a.m.: Citrus Magic or Lemon Ginger Turmeric Juice

11 a.m.: Super Ruby Greens

2 p.m.: The Emerald

5 p.m.: Super Ruby Greens

8 p.m.: Lemon Ginger Turmeric Juice

9 p.m.: Mint, Sleepytime, or chamomile tea

DAY 5

7 a.m.: Hot lemon in warm water or hot mint tea

8 a.m.: Lemon Ginger Turmeric Juice

11 a.m.: Super-Duper Juice

2 p.m.: Vital Greens

5 p.m.: Mineral Refresh

8 p.m.: The Stabilizer

9 p.m.: Mint, Sleepytime or chamomile tea

DAY 6

7 a.m.: Warm lemon water or hot mint tea

8 a.m.: Citrus Magic or Lemon Ginger Turmeric Juice

11 a.m.: Super Ruby Greens

2 p.m.: The Emerald

5 p.m.: Super Ruby Greens

8 p.m.: Lemon Ginger Turmeric Juice

9 p.m.: Mint, Sleepytime, or chamomile tea

DAY 7

7 a.m.: Warm lemon water or hot mint tea

8 a.m.: Lemon Ginger Turmeric Juice

11 a.m.: Super-Duper Juice

2 p.m.: Vital Greens

5 p.m.: Lemon Ginger Turmeric Juice

8 p.m.: The Stabilizer

9 p.m.: Mint, Sleepytime, or chamomile tea

ANGENIETA'S Story

I took a class on juicing from a nutritionist at the Center, and decided to do the 7-day juice fast. It ended up being the best fast that I've ever done in my life—and I've done many! In fact, I loved it so much that I ended up recommending and turning other people on to it.

The juices were tasty, and I was in a really good mood and felt amazing throughout the entire fast—almost euphoric, really. What's more, the recipe plan included both juices and smoothies, so I was never hungry. I would add avocado to some of the recipes, which made them more filling and taste great. If you do get hungry, you can add plant protein powder to the juices. Toward the end of the fast, I ate a couple of salads to ease out of it, and I really think that it did a lot to help me in my healing journey. While I am not on a fast now, every morning I continue to make smoothies from the vegetables that I grow in my garden.

In addition to juicing, I also follow a modified low-carbohydrate diet. Dr. Connealy discovered that I had precancerous cells due to mold toxicity. Also, my father had died at age fifty-eight of lung cancer, so she thought that I was at risk for developing it. The ketogenic diet was hard for me, but I have found that I can manage a low-carb diet if I don't have to be perfect and can occasionally eat things like an apple with almond butter. I found that it was more stressful for my body to try to do everything perfectly than to go off my diet occasionally, so I have continued to follow a healthy food plan but not be so strict with myself. And I think it is working!

CHAPTER 14

Living a Cancer-Free Life

IN THIS CHAPTER, YOU WILL FIND . . .

- A summary of wellness tools
- Testimonials from overcomers who have successfully used *The Cancer Revolution* tools
- A message of hope and encouragement

When you or somebody that you love has been diagnosed with cancer, it can be a frightening, scary, and emotionally tumultuous time. And what I'm going to say next may surprise you: Stay strong! Cancer doesn't need to be a "curtain call" but rather a "wake-up call"—an opportunity for you to reevaluate and re-create a better, healthier life for yourself. Most of us live in fear of cancer, but we don't need to because cancer isn't some mysterious force attacking the body and for which we have no answers.

An article published in the scientific journal *Pharmaceutical Research* suggests only 5 to 10 percent of all cancer cases are caused by genetic defects, whereas the remaining 90 to 95 percent may be caused by environmental and lifestyle factors, such as a poor diet, environmental pollutants, infections, stress, obesity, and physical inactivity.[1] This suggests we have the power to affect 90 to 95 percent of what causes cancer.

Unfortunately, conventional doctors are trained to treat their patients only with surgery, radiation, and chemotherapy. It's usually not standard that they seek out the root causes of disease that have allowed their patient's body to become a more favorable breeding ground for cancer. They don't look beyond the tumor or the cancer itself. Their focus is on the disease and not the whole person, and because of this, I feel the outcomes in conventional medicine are dismal.

But this doesn't have to be! Science has already provided us with the clues we need, and most integrative doctors take an approach based on that science. Our programs are well thought out and based on scientific studies, and my personal experience with many patients has illustrated this. Such treatments as hyperthermia, IV vitamin C, and SOT aren't fads; rather, they are supported by a plethora of studies and suggested by other doctors' experiences with their patients. Radical remission *can be* possible when you do these kinds of treatments, along with the other things I have shared with you in this book, including:

- Following a healthy food plan
- Detoxifying your body and home, and removing the junk that may have caused your body to become sick in the first place
- Balancing your body's chemistry with nutritional supplements, herbs, bioidentical hormones, and other remedies
- Exercising regularly
- Practicing stress-reduction techniques
- Getting deep, restful sleep every night
- Putting together a support system, which includes finding skilled, successful, and experienced integrative cancer doctor(s)

Chemotherapy and radiation have their place in treatment, but I feel they are simply not enough because cancer isn't caused by one thing but by a plethora of different things, and we must address all of these things, not just the tumor. This is nonnegotiable because your goal is to create a healthy body, and you need all of the tools that we share in this book to help do that. You must pull out every thorn that has helped cause your body to become a hospitable place for disease, and create balance in every organ, tissue, and system.

Don't feel that you need to do everything perfectly, though. If you can't do a 7-day juice fast, or exercise every single day, or follow your diet to a T—that's okay! Even if you used just one of the tools in this book, it could help you tremendously. At the same time, it's the magical combination of doing all of these things together, and rotating treatments, that helps create the recipe for success.

So, we encourage you to do what you can; just start somewhere, and add something new to your regimen every week, realizing that you want to eventually address every cause of disease with all of the tools that we've provided in this book. Because the more you are able to do, the more you will be helping to change your internal terrain so your body becomes a less hospitable place for disease.

To further encourage you, I'd just like to share a couple more patient success stories with you. These are patients who, perhaps like you, once had no hope but found it being restored once they realized that there was a new, better road they could take in their wellness journey. Let their stories speak to your heart and mind, and embrace them, as you might find the seeds for your own wellness within their words.

Elizabeth, a forty-five-year-old married woman from the Midwest, was diagnosed with stage 4 breast cancer two years ago and told by her conventional doctors that there was little that could be done for her. But two years later, she is feeling great and is optimistic about her recovery. She had a mastectomy, followed by numerous integrative treatments at our clinic, including insulin potentiation targeted low-dose chemotherapy (IPTLD) and SOT (supportive oligonucleotide technique) treatment. In addition, she regularly detoxifies her body, uses a hyperbaric oxygen chamber (which she purchased for at-home use), and has made dramatic lifestyle and dietary changes. Her key advice for those who want to beat cancer is: "Eat as though your life depended upon it. Make sure to detoxify your liver. Avoid sugar and processed foods. Eat lots of vegetables and choose organic foods."

Maria is another patient whose story is a shining example of how staying the course and following a holistic wellness regimen can benefit the body. A fifty-six-year-old divorced mother of four, Maria found a tiny lump in her breast the morning after her fifty-fourth birthday, almost three years ago. Although her mammogram just six months prior had been completely clear, a biopsy revealed she had an aggressive type of breast cancer. So, Maria had the tumor removed, and when her blood work came back and showed that the cancer had not spread, she decided not to pursue high-dose chemotherapy and radiation, despite her second surgeon having recommended that she do so.

Maria was led to our clinic, where she received a variety of intensive IV treatments. Her health is now improved, but she works hard to maintain it. She detoxifies her body regularly with liver cleanses, and walks for thirty minutes daily. She also maintains a healthy diet, and takes a variety of supplements linked with cancer prevention. She avoids sugar, gets a good night's sleep every night, and deals with stress by writing in a journal.

And then there's my own health. Although I am at high risk for developing cancer genetically speaking, I've successfully avoided it. I'm now in my fifth decade of life and my health is outstanding because I practice what I preach and I live out the principles I have shared with you in this book.

Once you have a vision and understand your condition, you have a greater chance of changing your condition. It is possible to fight and prevent cancer, but you must be dedicated to your wellness process, and believe in yourself and in those whom you have chosen to be on your support system, and use the tools I have shared throughout *The Cancer Revolution*. Once you do these things, and experience the benefits of this approach, I hope you will want to start your own "cancer revolution" and share this book with others. Indeed, if every one of us, including every doctor, took the time to learn about and educate others about the possibilities, we could help win the war against cancer on a global scale, and witness not only ourselves, but also more of our family, friends, and society living healthy, vibrant, cancer-free lives.

The Recipes:
Dishes for Repairing and
Restoring Your Body

Here you will learn how to create delicious, nutritious, anticancer salads, soups, entrées, snacks, desserts, and beverages based on the food plan guidelines outlined in Chapter 4. Created by our nutritionist, Liliana Partida (www.LilianaPartida.com), these recipes are compatible with most low-carb food plans, including the ketogenic diet.

The Anticancer Kitchen

Most of the recipes that you'll find here can be prepared using tools and ingredients that are commonly found in most kitchens and at your local grocery store. However, a few require specialty tools or ingredients that are not listed in Chapter 4. Following is a list of those items, which you may want to add to your shopping list.

Ingredients

These items can be found at your local health food store (e.g., Trader Joe's, Ralph's, or Whole Foods), and/or at many online retailers. Most can also be found at your local grocery store, although you may find a wider selection at a health food store.

Almond meal
Bragg Liquid Aminos
Celtic sea salt
Chia seeds
Coconut amino acids
Coconut flour
Curry paste
Fresh wheatgrass products (e.g., Mega Greens)
Hemp seeds
Kefir (organic fermented cow's milk)
MCT (medium-chain triglyceride) liquid coconut oil
Nut milks (e.g., almond)
Nutritional yeast
Pine nuts
Pumpkin seeds
Raw cacao or cacao nibs
Stevia
Sugarless chocolate protein powder (e.g., PlantFusion)
Whey- or plant-based protein powder

We recommend any/all of the following protein powder products (see Resources for product website information):

Nutiva Hemp Protein
PlantFusion (NutraFusion Nutritionals)
Reserveage Organics Grass-Fed Whey Protein
Sunwarrior Warrior Blend Raw Vegan Protein
Super Protein in the Buff (Boku Superfoods)
TerasWhey Organic Whey Protein

Tools

You can purchase the following items at most department and domestic merchandise stores throughout the United States. They can also be purchased at large online retailers, such as Amazon.com and eBay.com.

Cheesecloth (optional, for nut milk recipes)
Dehydrator (optional, for dehydrating nuts, seeds, and vegetables)
Immersion blender
Juicer (for the juices in the 7-day plan)
Nut milk bag (optional, for nut milk recipes)
Salad spinner (optional, to dry lettuce/kale)
Vegetable spiralizer
Vegetable steamer
Vitamix (for the blended juices and smoothies in this section)

Fresh Blender Juices

Spicy Green
Ginger Snap
Simply Greens Detox Beverage
Sweet Greens
Fresh Veggie Juice
Protein Powder Veggie Juice
Fresh Gazpacho Blender Juice
Ginger Lemon Drink
Mega Greens Drink
Apple Drink

Drinking vegetables is a great way for your body to quickly receive vital phytonutrients, since the vegetables are absorbed into your bloodstream within fifteen minutes after you drink the juice. These phytonutrients energize, detoxify, and alkalinize you. Chapter 13 outlined a 7-day juicing cleanse; you can also use those recipes as a basis for blender (rather than juicer) drinks. Unlike the recipes in Chapter 13, the recipes in this section are all made with a high-speed blender, rather than a juicer. A high-speed blender gives you a smoother juice than a regular blender or food processor can. If you do not use a high-speed blender, you may need to blend in batches, especially with more fibrous produce.

Some tips to get the most out of your juice:

- Make sure that the vegetables that you use are organic, fresh, and well washed. If your produce is not organic, be sure to remove the peel before using it.
- It is best to consume green drinks by themselves, without other foods. Wait at least a half-hour before consuming other foods to get the best benefits from juicing.
- You can also add a scoop of protein powder to any of the following juices and use the juice as a meal replacement, or take Master Amino Acid Pattern (MAP) capsules as a protein substitute thirty minutes before the juice.

To make all the following juices, simply combine the ingredients in a blender. Each recipe makes about 16 ounces of juice, or one serving. It's best to drink the juices within an hour. If needed, you can store them in the refrigerator for up to 24 hours, but to retain the nutrients and enzymes, you should drink them right away.

Spicy Green

3 celery stalks
1 carrot, trimmed
1 cucumber, peeled

Handful of fresh parsley
1 (dime-size) slice fresh ginger, peeled, or to taste (optional)

Ginger Snap

3 celery stalks
1 cup Swiss chard leaves
1 lemon, peeled and seeded
1 (quarter-size) slice fresh ginger, peeled, or to taste (optional)

½ cucumber, peeled
Handful of fresh parsley
1 scoop plant-based protein powder, or ½ avocado (optional)

Simply Greens Detox Beverage

1 cucumber, peeled
Handful of fresh parsley
Handful of Swiss chard
Handful of spinach

1 (quarter-size) slice fresh ginger, peeled
1 lemon, peeled and seeded
2 carrots, trimmed

Sweet Greens

Handful of spinach
1 cucumber, peeled

1 carrot, trimmed
3 celery stalks

Fresh Veggie Juice

1 tomato, seeded
1 cucumber, peeled
½ red bell pepper, seeded
2 tablespoons chopped onion

Pinch of cayenne pepper
Handful of fresh Italian parsley
1 cup purified water, or to taste
1 teaspoon olive oil

Protein Powder Veggie Juice

1 cup Swiss chard
1 cucumber, peeled
3 celery stalks
1 lemon, peeled and seeded
Handful of fresh parsley

2 to 3 cups purified water, or to taste
Stevia, to taste
½ scoop plant-based protein powder
    (optional)

Fresh Gazpacho Blender Juice

½ red bell pepper, seeded
1 cucumber, peeled
1 tomato, seeded
1 to 2 tablespoons chopped
    onion

Handful of fresh parsley or spinach
1 carrot
Pinch of cayenne pepper

Ginger Lemon Drink

Stevia, to taste
1 lemon, peeled and seeded
1 (quarter-size) slice fresh
    ginger, peeled, or to taste

10 ounces purified water

Mega Greens Drink

This is a simple yet powerful wheatgrass drink; one that you'll have regularly on the 14-day plan.

 1 to 2 scoops Mega Green wheatgrass powder
 16 ounces purified water

Stir the powder into the water with a spoon or combine in a blender.

Apple Drink

This refreshing tonic is especially helpful to remedy constipation.

 1 small organic apple, cored and seeded,
    or ¼ cup freshly pressed apple juice
 1 to 2 ounces aloe vera juice
 1 to 2 tablespoons psyllium husks

Create Your Own Juice Recipes

You can also create your own juices by combining vegetables from the following list of ingredients. Use vegetables that have strong flavors and powerful anticancer properties, such as parsley and garlic, in small amounts; no more than 1 to 2 garlic cloves per drink, and no more than ½ cup of fresh parsley per drink. To these, you can add one or two bitter vegetables, such as spinach, kale, or another dark leafy green—1 to 2 cups per 8-ounce beverage. You might then add half of a cucumber and up to four celery stalks to make a nice base for the drink. If you aren't following a ketogenic or strict low-glycemic diet, you could also add a carrot. Finally, adding stevia, fresh ginger, or lemon to any of these juices can go a long way toward offsetting the flavors of the bitter greens and making them more palatable. (Note: Dark leafy greens should be used in small amounts if you have thyroid problems or your doctor advises you to stay away from dark leafy greens that contain the mineral molybdenum.)

Prime Fruits and Vegetables for Juicing

These fruits and vegetables benefit or support the following health conditions and/or organs:

Cabbage—colitis, ulcers

Carrots—eyes, arthritis, osteoporosis

Celery—kidneys, diabetes, osteoporosis

Cilantro—removes heavy metals

Cucumber—edema, diabetes

Garlic—allergies, colds, hypertension, cardiovascular disease, fatty liver, diabetes

Ginger—anti-inflammatory, antimicrobial

Greens (kale, collards, chard, etc.)—cardiovascular disease, skin and digestive problems, eczema, obesity, and bad breath

Jerusalem artichokes—diabetes

Lemon—liver, gallbladder, allergies, asthma, cardiovascular disease, and colds

Parsley—kidneys, liver, supports immunity

Radish—fatty liver, obesity

Spinach—anemia, eczema

Turmeric—anti-inflammatory

Watercress—anemia, liver, intestines, bad breath

Nut Milks and Protein Powder Drinks

Basic Homemade Nut Milk
Mocha Nut Milk Shake
Coco Loco Nut Shake
Whey or Plant Protein Powder Drink

For the following drinks, you can use either store-bought or homemade nut milk. We prefer homemade nut milk since it is free of artificial fillers, sugar, or caseinates. Nut milks are a superior option to soy milk because all soy products, even those that are GMO-free, are cooked and difficult for the body to digest.

Basic Homemade Nut Milk

This basic nut milk recipe calls for almonds, but you can substitute any nut or seed (or a combination of seeds) to make the milk. You can drink the milk straight, use it in other drink or smoothie recipes, or use as a substitute in recipes that call for dairy milk. If you prefer a sweeter taste, you can add stevia and/or vanilla extract.

Makes 4 servings
>4 cups purified water
>1 cup raw organic almonds or other nuts
>Stevia (optional)
>Pure vanilla extract (optional)

Fill an 8- to 9-inch baking pan with 2 cups of the water, then add the nuts. Soak overnight, or for a minimum of 8 hours or a maximum of twelve, then rinse and drain the nuts.

Place the nuts and the remaining 2 cups of water in a blender and blend until smooth. Add the stevia and/or vanilla to taste, if using. If you prefer a very smooth drink, you can strain the milk with a fine-mesh strainer, through several layers of cheesecloth, or with a nut milk bag. Nut milk will keep in the refrigerator for up to 3 days.

Mocha Nut Milk Shake

Makes 1 serving
>3 tablespoons hemp seeds
>2 tablespoons chia seeds
>1 tablespoon raw cacao or cacao nibs (optional)
>1 cup unsweetened almond, hemp, or coconut milk
>Stevia

Place the ingredients in a high-speed blender, adding the stevia to taste. Add four or five ice cubes and blend the ingredients together for 30 seconds to 1 minute on high speed. Serve and enjoy. Best consumed within an hour.

Coco Loco Nut Shake

Makes 1 serving

3 tablespoons hemp seeds

2 tablespoons chia seeds

1 cup unsweetened almond,
   hemp, or coconut milk

1 tablespoon coconut oil

Ground cinnamon

Pure vanilla extract

Stevia

Place the ingredients in a high-speed blender, adding the cinnamon, vanilla, and stevia to taste. Add four or five ice cubes. Blend the ingredients together for 30 seconds to 1 minute on high speed. Serve and enjoy. Best consumed within an hour.

Whey or Plant Protein Powder Drink

Makes 1 serving

1 to 2 scoops plant-based protein powder (see page 226)

1 cup unsweetened almond milk

1 tablespoon chia seeds

2 tablespoons coconut oil

Stevia

Place the ingredients in a blender, adding stevia to taste. Blend the ingredients together for 30 seconds to 1 minute on high speed. Serve and enjoy. Best consumed within an hour.

Basic Beverages

Lemon/Limeade

Iced Green Tea

Anti-Inflammatory Tea

Fiber Drink

Cider Vinegar Drink

Savory Sipping Alkaline Broth

Lemon/Limeade

Makes 4 servings

1 to 2 lemons

32 ounces still purified or
    sparkling water

Stevia

4 lemon wedges

Using a lemon press, extract the juice from the lemons, then add the juice
to the water. Sweeten to taste with stevia. Add the lemon wedges and
serve. The lemonade can be stored in the refrigerator for 3 to 5 days.

Iced Green Tea

Makes 4 servings

3 or 4 organic green or herbal
    tea bags

1 cup boiling purified water

24 ounces cool purified water

Stevia

Place the tea bags in the boiling water and let them steep for 2 minutes. Pour
the tea into a 32-ounce mason jar and top up with the cool water. Add
ice or refrigerate the tea. Sweeten to taste with Stevia. The tea will keep in
the refrigerator for 3 to 5 days.

Note: If you are sensitive to caffeine, steep the tea for just 2 minutes, dump
the first brew, then add boiling filtered water to the tea bags again and
steep for a second time. By the second brew, most of the caffeine will
be gone.

Anti-Inflammatory Tea

Makes 3 servings

1 (4-inch) piece organic fresh
    ginger, sliced diagonally
    into small pieces

1 (4-inch) piece organic fresh
    turmeric, sliced diago-
    nally into small pieces

6¼ cups (50 ounces) purified water

Juice of 2 lemons

Stevia

Place the ginger, turmeric, and purified water in a large saucepan and bring to a boil. Boil for 5 minutes. Turn off the heat and let the mixture steep for 5 hours. Strain the tea, discarding the roots. Add the lemon juice to the tea, along with stevia to taste. Store the tea in the refrigerator in three 16-ounce mason jars for up to 3 days.

Fiber Drink

This drink is an easy way to add more fiber to your diet. The cinnamon and stevia make a light, sweetly spicy taste. Make sure to drink it immediately, or the liquid will thicken.

Makes 1 serving

1 teaspoon psyllium husks

¼ teaspoon ground cinnamon (optional)

8 ounces purified water

Stevia (optional)

Combine the psyllium, cinnamon, and water in a large glass. Add stevia to taste, if using. Stir with a spoon and consume immediately.

Cider Vinegar Drink

Makes 1 serving

1 teaspoon organic cider vinegar

8 ounces purified water

Stevia (optional)

Stir the cider vinegar into the water. Add stevia to taste, if using.

Savory Sipping Alkaline Broth

Makes 6 servings

2 cups green beans

2 cups celery, chopped into 2-inch pieces

2 cups zucchini, chopped into 2-inch pieces

6 to 8 cups purified water

Place the vegetables and water in a medium-size saucepan and bring to a boil. Boil for 30 minutes. Strain the liquid, discarding the vegetables. The broth will keep in the refrigerator for 3 days, and can also be frozen.

Fast and Easy Breakfasts

The following fast, easy-to-make breakfast recipes are designed to jump-start your metabolism and stabilize your blood sugar. They are high in protein and should keep you satiated for hours.

Poached Eggs
Hard-Boiled Eggs
Turkey Bacon

Poached Eggs

Makes 1 serving

Olive oil or coconut spray
2 or 3 large eggs

1 cup purified water

Spray a 6-inch skillet with olive oil spray. Heat the skillet, then crack all the eggs together into the skillet and cover with a lid for 30 seconds. When you see that the eggs are starting to bubble, add the water to the skillet, replace the lid, and cook until the eggs reach your desired consistency. For a nice soft center, cook the eggs for about 2 minutes. Remove from the skillet and serve immediately.

Hard-Boiled Eggs

Makes 2 servings

1 teaspoon aluminum-free baking soda
4 large eggs
2 to 3 cups purified water

Fill a 1-quart saucepan with water. Add the baking soda. Bring the water to a boil, then lower the heat to a simmer, add the eggs, and cook for 10 minutes. Remove the pan from the heat, drain the water, and immediately place 1 cup of ice cubes in the pan, along with 2 to 3 cups of cold water, and let sit for 10 minutes, or until the eggs are completely cooled.

Break off a tiny portion of the shell at either end of an egg, using your fingernail. Hold the egg in your hand and blow into one side of the egg. When you do this, the shell will break, and if you are lucky, the egg will pop right out of the shell. (So, be prepared to catch it!) Repeat with the other eggs. The eggs can be stored in the refrigerator for up to 3 days.

Turkey Bacon

Makes 2 servings

Coconut or olive oil spray
4 turkey bacon strips (nitrate- and sugar-free)

Coat a 6-inch skillet with coconut oil spray. Place the bacon strips flat in the pan and cook over medium heat until the strips are browned, or about 2 minutes. Turkey bacon can be stored in the refrigerator for up to 3 days.

Dips, Sauces, and Marinades

These delicious recipes add savory flavor to any meat or vegetable dish and provide a satisfying finish to your entrées and sides. They are creamy, rich, and filling and contain healing herbs, amino acids, and metabolically friendly fats that provide essential nutrition to the body. Suggestions for their use are listed throughout the Recipes.

Fresh Mayonnaise
MCT Metabolically Friendly Mayonnaise
Spicy Burger Sauce
Fresh Salsa
Fresh Guacamole
Tomato and Basil Topping
Parsley Pesto
Pine Nut or Walnut Dip

Curry Sauce
Creamy Curry Dip
Dijon Chicken Marinade
Lamb or Beef Marinade
Italian Marinade
Teriyaki Marinade
Asian Marinade
Ginger Citrus Marinade

Fresh Mayonnaise

This recipe is a great substitute for ketchup, mustard, and/or traditional mayonnaise over hamburgers and turkey burgers, because unlike these traditional sauces, it contains no sugar, soy, harmful fats, or additives or preservatives. This recipe can also be used as a dip for carrots and celery.

Makes 3 cups mayonnaise
   2 organic large egg yolks
   1 large egg
   1 tablespoon gluten-free Dijon mustard
   Celtic sea salt
   ¼ cup freshly squeezed lemon juice
   1½ to 2 cups nut or seed oil or light olive oil
   Fresh garlic, basil, tarragon, and/or dill (optional)

Blend together the egg yolks, egg, mustard, a pinch of the salt, and half of the lemon juice in a blender or food processor at medium speed for 1 minute. With the motor still running, drizzle the oil into the blender in a slow steady stream, until the mixture reaches your desired consistency. Taste the mixture and add more lemon juice, if desired. Season to taste with additional Celtic sea salt and garlic and/or herbs. The mayonnaise keeps in a glass container in the refrigerator for up to 5 days. Allow it to return to room temperature before stirring and using.

MCT Metabolically Friendly Mayonnaise

This recipe contains MCT oil, an anticancer oil that promotes a healthy metabolism and which lowers inflammation. It can also be used as a dip for carrots and celery.

Makes about 1 cup mayonnaise, or 8 servings
  1 large egg
  ½ teaspoon gluten-free Dijon mustard
  1 tablespoon freshly squeezed lemon juice
  Pinch of Celtic sea salt
  1 cup MCT liquid coconut oil
  Fresh garlic, basil, tarragon, and/or dill

Place all the ingredients in a wide-mouthed mason jar. Let the coconut oil rise to the top. Place an immersion blender at the bottom of the jar and turn on. As the mayo emulsifies, slowly raise the immersion blender out of the jar and pulse it a few times until the whole mixture is thick and creamy. Season to taste with additional Celtic sea salt, garlic, and herbs. The mayo will keep in the refrigerator for up to 2 weeks.

Spicy Burger Sauce

This tasty sauce can be used over hamburgers, turkey burgers, lettuce-wrapped fish tacos, and baked chicken. It's also great drizzled over steamed vegetables, such as Brussels sprouts, zucchini, and asparagus.

Makes ½ cup sauce, or enough for 4 burgers
  ½ cup organic or homemade mayonnaise (page 238)
  1 teaspoon chipotle hot sauce, or to taste
  ¼ teaspoon dried dill
  1 teaspoon freshly squeezed lemon juice

Whisk all the ingredients together in a medium-size bowl. The sauce can be stored in the refrigerator for up to 4 days.

Fresh Salsa

This salsa tastes great drizzled over turkey taco and chicken lettuce wraps, as well as over hamburgers and meat loaf.

Makes about 1 cup salsa, or about 4 servings

4 cups purified water

4 large tomatoes

1 garlic clove, finely minced

1 ounce mild green chile, or
1 to 2 tablespoons
minced fresh hot chile or
jalapeño pepper

½ cup minced green onion or onion

¼ cup chopped fresh cilantro, or to
taste

1 teaspoon freshly squeezed lime or
lemon juice

1 teaspoon Celtic sea salt, or to taste

In 3-quart soup pot, bring the water to a boil. Meanwhile, make a crisscross cut across the top of the tomatoes, using a knife. This makes it easy to remove the tomatoes' skin after they are blanched. Blanch the tomatoes in the boiling water for 1 minute, or until the skin pulls away from the crisscross area at the top of the tomatoes. Make sure not to overcook the tomatoes. Using tongs, remove the tomatoes from the water and peel off the skin. Then, chop the tomatoes into ¼-inch pieces and discard the seeds, reserving the juice. Mix the pieces together in a bowl, along with the garlic, chile, green onion, cilantro, citrus juice, salt, and the juice from the tomatoes. The salsa will keep in the refrigerator for up to 4 days.

Fresh Guacamole

Guacamole can be used as a dip for celery, carrots, cucumbers, and other raw veggies, as well as a garnish for turkey tacos.

Makes about 1 cup guacamole, or about 4 servings

2 avocados, peeled and pitted

1 tomato

2 green onions, chopped

1 garlic clove

Juice of 1 lemon

¼ teaspoon Celtic sea salt

Cayenne pepper or powdered
chipotle seasoning (optional)

Fresh cilantro

In a small bowl, mash the avocados with a fork and set aside. Chop the tomato into small pieces, draining off any excess water. Add the tomato to the avocado, along with the chopped green onions, and stir to combine. Crush the garlic in a garlic press and add to the mixture, along with the lemon juice and the salt. Add the cayenne and cilantro to taste, if using. Store any leftovers in the refrigerator and consume within 24 hours. If you put an avocado pit into the guacamole, it will help keep the guacamole from turning brown over time.

Tomato and Basil Topping

This topping is delicious drizzled over zucchini or eggplant, or any type of meat, such as chicken or beef.

Makes 4 servings

4 cups purified water	1 tablespoon tomato paste
3 tomatoes	1 teaspoon Celtic sea salt
½ cup chopped fresh basil	Pinch of cayenne pepper, or to taste
1 tablespoon olive oil	1 teaspoon cayenne seasoning,
4 garlic cloves	or to taste

In 3-quart soup pot, bring the water to a boil. Meanwhile, make a crisscross cut across the top of the tomatoes, using a knife. This makes it easy to remove the tomatoes' skin after they are blanched. Blanch the tomatoes in the boiling water for 1 minute, or until the skin pulls away from the crisscross area at the top of the tomatoes. Make sure not to overcook the tomatoes. Using tongs, remove the tomatoes from the water and peel off the skin. Chop the tomatoes into small cubes, removing the seeds as you go.

Place the tomatoes in a small bowl and mix in the basil. Set the bowl aside.

Pour the olive oil into a 1-quart saucepan and sauté the garlic over low heat. Add the tomato mixture and tomato paste, and cook for 5 to 8 minutes. Add the salt, cayenne, and cayenne seasoning to taste. The sauce will keep in the refrigerator for 2 to 4 days.

Parsley Pesto

This dairy-free pesto is an excellent sauce to use over Zucchini Noodles (page 271) or chicken.

Makes ¾ cup pesto

½ cup raw pine nuts or
    walnuts
¼ to ⅓ cup olive oil
1 tablespoon purified water

3 to 4 garlic cloves
1 to 2 cups fresh parsley
1 tablespoon freshly squeezed
    lemon juice

Place all the ingredients in a blender and blend on medium speed until smooth. The sauce will keep in the refrigerator for at least a week.

Pine Nut or Walnut Dip

This recipe uses pine nuts, rather than a dairy product, as a thickening agent. The dip can be used as a mayonnaise or dip for veggies, to thicken soups, as an addition to smoothies, and over Cinnamon Chia Pudding (page 282). The cream portion of the recipe can also be used as a thickening agent in any recipe that calls for cream.

Makes about ½ cup dip

1 cup organic pine nuts or
    walnuts
2½ cups purified water
1 teaspoon rice vinegar
1 teaspoon coconut amino
    acids
1 teaspoon sesame oil

1 tablespoon olive oil
2 to 3 roasted or fresh garlic cloves
½ teaspoon grated fresh ginger
Cayenne pepper
Celtic sea salt
1 drop of stevia, or to taste
1 tablespoon toasted sesame seeds

Soak the pine nuts in 2 cups of the water in the refrigerator overnight or for
    8 hours.
Drain the liquid and place the nuts in a blender, then add the remaining
    ½ cup of water, and blend until the mixture reaches a whipped cream–

like consistency. Add the rice vinegar and coconut amino acids and blend together on medium speed. Slowly drizzle in the sesame and olive oil, then the garlic, and blend again. Add the ginger, cayenne, salt, stevia, if using, and the sesame seeds. Continue to blend the ingredients together until the dip easily coats the back of a spoon. Chill for 20 minutes or longer. Store in a glass container in the refrigerator for up to 4 days.

Curry Sauce

This curry is flavorful without being too spicy. You can cook any meat, such as fish or chicken, or vegetables in the curry at the same time that you are cooking the curry.

Makes about 4 servings

1 teaspoon coconut oil	1 tablespoon coconut amino acids
1 tablespoon gluten-free red curry paste	½ teaspoon lime zest
1 teaspoon grated fresh ginger	1 serrano or Thai chile (optional)
1 cup thick organic coconut milk	15 fresh basil leaves, chopped

Heat the coconut oil in a medium-size saucepan. Add the curry paste and ginger and briefly fry the ingredients together over medium heat. Add the remaining ingredients. Stirring the mixture well, simmer for 5 minutes, taking care not to boil it. The sauce can be stored in the refrigerator for up to 3 days.

To use: Cut two 3- to 4-ounce raw chicken breasts or fish fillets into 1-inch pieces and place them in the sauce. Simmer the entire mixture for another 5 to 6 minutes.

Creamy Curry Dip

This is a flavorful dip for raw vegetables, such as asparagus, zucchini, and green beans. It can also be used as a sandwich spread. Serve over raw veggies on a platter for a filling meal. The dip can also be drizzled over hot vegetables.

Makes ½ cup dip, or about 4 servings
- ½ cup organic or homemade mayonnaise (page 238)
- Squirt of freshly squeezed lemon juice
- ½ teaspoon coconut amino acids
- ½ teaspoon curry powder
- ½ teaspoon ground turmeric
- ¼ teaspoon ground cumin

Whisk all the ingredients together in a bowl. Chill in the refrigerator for an hour, then serve. The dip can be stored in the refrigerator for up to 1 week.

Dijon Chicken Marinade

This marinade pairs well with boneless, skinless chicken breasts. It is a great accompaniment to a baby green side salad and/or cooked broccoli, green beans, or asparagus.

Makes 4 servings
- Juice of ½ lemon
- 1 tablespoon grainy gluten-free Dijon mustard
- 2 tablespoons olive oil
- 2 garlic cloves
- 1 tablespoon coconut amino acids
- 1 teaspoon Italian or tarragon seasoning

Whisk the lemon juice and mustard together in a small bowl. Drizzle in the olive oil, then press in the garlic, using a garlic press. Add the remaining ingredients. The marinade can be stored in the refrigerator for 3 to 4 days.

To use: Cut two 3- to 4-ounce raw chicken breasts into 1-inch pieces. Marinate the chicken in the mixture for 30 minutes to 1 hour before broiling.

Lamb or Beef Marinade

This marinade is delicious served over broiled lamb or beef. You can also soak uncooked lamb or beef in it for thirty minutes prior to cooking, to give the meat a more savory flavor.

Makes about 4 servings

2 tablespoons fresh rosemary, chopped
2 tablespoons chopped fresh or dried mint
2 to 4 garlic cloves, chopped
1 tablespoon red wine vinegar
1 teaspoon balsamic vinegar
2 to 4 tablespoons olive oil
2 tablespoons coconut amino acids or tamari sauce
Celtic sea salt

Whisk together all the ingredients, except the salt, in a small bowl. Add salt to taste. The marinade can be stored in the refrigerator for 3 to 4 days.

Italian Marinade

This marinade is great for boneless, skinless broiled chicken breasts.

Makes about 4 servings

Juice of ½ lemon
2 to 4 garlic cloves, pressed
1 tablespoon grainy gluten-free Dijon mustard
1 teaspoon Italian or tarragon seasoning
2 to 3 tablespoons olive oil
Celtic sea salt

Whisk all the ingredients together in a small bowl, then let the mixture sit for 30 minutes. The marinade can be stored in the refrigerator for 3 to 4 days.

To use: Cut two 3- to 4-ounce raw chicken breasts into 1-inch pieces. Marinate the chicken in the mixture for 30 minutes to 1 hour before broiling.

Teriyaki Marinade

Soak your seafood, lamb, or other red meat, and/or chicken in this marinade before cooking it. The marinade is also delicious as a sauce drizzled over these same meats.

Makes about 4 servings

Juice of ½ lemon

1 tablespoon grated or pressed fresh ginger

2 tablespoons coconut amino acids

Zest of ¼ orange, along with 1 tablespoon freshly squeezed orange juice

2 garlic cloves, pressed or finely chopped

Stevia (optional)

2 to 3 tablespoons olive oil

Whisk all the ingredients together in a small bowl, then let the meat soak in the mixture for 30 minutes. You can also spread the marinade over already broiled steak, seafood, or chicken, if you prefer, and use it as a sauce. Store in the refrigerator for up to 4 days.

Asian Marinade

This marinade is ideal drizzled over the Seared Toasted Sesame Salmon Salad (page 258). You can also marinate uncooked fish or chicken in it, or pour it over any kind of broiled or baked fish or chicken.

Makes ½ cup marinade, or 4 servings

Juice of ½ lemon

1 (½- to 1-inch) piece fresh ginger, grated or pressed

¼ cup gluten-free coconut amino acids

2 tablespoons olive oil

1 tablespoon sesame oil

½ teaspoon orange zest

2 to 3 garlic cloves, pressed or finely chopped

1 teaspoon toasted sesame seeds

Whisk all the ingredients together in a bowl, then marinate your choice of chicken or fish in the mixture for 30 minutes to 1 hour. The marinade can be stored in the refrigerator for 3 to 4 days.

Ginger Citrus Marinade

This marinade is delicious over Seared Toasted Sesame Salmon Salad (page 258), or baked chicken or broiled steak.

Makes ¼ cup marinade, or about 2 servings

Juice of ½ lemon

1 teaspoon grated fresh ginger

3 to 4 garlic cloves, pressed

Celtic sea salt

1 drop of stevia (optional)

2 tablespoons olive oil

Whisk all the ingredients together in a bowl, seasoning to taste with the ginger, salt, and stevia, if using. Spread over broiled or baked steak, fish, or chicken. Alternatively, marinate the meat for 30 minutes in the mixture before cooking. Store the marinade in the refrigerator for up to 4 days.

Salads and Salad Dressings

Build your meals around your green salads, which provide alkalinizing and live enzymes to the body, along with fiber, water, vitamins, minerals, and vital phytonutrients. This section contains recipes for both side and entrée salads. You can pair any of the following side salads with any side dish or entrée in the Recipes, or consume the entrée salads as a stand-alone meal. For optimal health and digestion, eat a salad at least once daily. Add to your salads any of the salad dressing recipes in this section, which are an excellent source of EFAs and amino acids and essential for rebuilding the body.

Dressings
MCT Essential Salad Dressing
French Salad Dressing
Citrus Delight Dressing
Cilantro Salad Dressing
Basil Salad Dressing
Creamy Garlic Dressing
Caesar Salad Dressing

Hearty Salads
Baby Greens Side Salad
Arugula Side Salad
Kale Side Salad
Greek Side Salad
Nutty Greek Salad
Greek Salad with Chicken
Chinese Chicken Salad
Curry Chicken Salad
Chicken Caesar Salad
Ceviche Salad
Seared Toasted Sesame Salmon Salad
Salmon Salad with Avocado
Sautéed Scallops Seafood Salad

The salads and dressings in this section are all light, healthy, easy to make—and tasty. If you don't wish to make salad dressing, you can simply add MCT liquid coconut oil, olive oil, salsa, or just a spray of coconut amino acids and lemon to your salads. Also consider adding garlic, for its anticancer properties.

The following dressings are delicious with most green side salads: romaine lettuce, baby greens, butter leaf lettuce, or spinach.

Dressings

MCT Essential Salad Dressing

Makes up to 6 servings

6 tablespoons MCT liquid coconut or olive oil

Juice of ½ lemon

½ teaspoon coconut amino acids

1 tablespoon gluten-free Dijon mustard (optional)

1 to 2 garlic cloves, pressed

Whisk all the ingredients together in a small bowl until they are fully combined. Store in a glass container in the refrigerator for up to 4 days.

French Salad Dressing

Makes up to 6 servings

1 tablespoon gluten-free Dijon mustard

Juice of ½ lemon

6 tablespoons olive oil

Purified water (optional)

1 to 2 garlic cloves, pressed

Dried tarragon

Celtic sea salt

Stevia (optional)

Whisk the mustard and lemon juice together in a small bowl. Slowly drizzle in the olive oil and whisk until the mixture thickens. If it gets too thick, add a bit of purified water. Whisk in the remaining ingredients, adding the tarragon, salt, and stevia, if using, to taste. Taste. If the dressing is too tart, add a bit more oil. Store in a glass container in the refrigerator for up to 4 days.

Citrus Delight Dressing

Makes up to 6 servings

6 tablespoons MCT liquid coconut or olive oil
Juice of ½ lemon
½ teaspoon coconut amino acids
Grated fresh ginger
Celtic sea salt
Stevia

Whisk all the ingredients together in a small bowl, adding the ginger, salt, and stevia to taste. Store in a glass container in the refrigerator for up to 4 days.

Cilantro Salad Dressing

Makes up to 6 servings

6 tablespoons MCT liquid coconut or olive oil
Juice of ½ lemon
1 teaspoon gluten-free Dijon mustard
½ teaspoon coconut amino acids
1 to 2 garlic cloves, crushed
2 tablespoons purified water
Pinch of cayenne pepper (optional)
Celtic sea salt
Handful of fresh cilantro
½ avocado

Whisk together all the ingredients, except the cilantro and avocado, in a bowl, adding cayenne to taste. Pour half of the mixture into a blender, and blend on medium to high speed for a minute. Add the avocado and cilantro, and blend until the mixture is thick and smooth. Add the blended mixture to the remaining dressing in the bowl and stir with a spoon. Store in a glass jar. The dressing will keep in the refrigerator for up to 4 days.

Basil Salad Dressing

Makes 6 servings

Juice of ½ lemon
1 teaspoon gluten-free Dijon mustard (optional)
⅓ cup MCT liquid coconut or olive oil
1 teaspoon liquid amino acids
1 to 2 garlic cloves, minced
Celtic sea salt
½ avocado, diced
Handful of fresh basil and/or parsley, minced
2 tablespoons purified water
Stevia (optional)

Whisk the lemon juice and mustard together in a small bowl. Drizzle in the
oil until the mixture coats the back of a spoon. Add the amino acids,
garlic, and salt to taste.

Pour half of the mixture into a blender, and blend on medium to high speed
for a minute. Add the avocado, basil, and water and blend until smooth,
adding stevia to taste, if using. Pour the mixture back into the remaining dressing. Store in a glass jar in the refrigerator for up to 4 days.

Creamy Garlic Dressing

*This dressing is delicious drizzled over the Salmon Salad (page 259), as well as
over shredded raw cabbage. It can also be served over cooked shrimp or chicken.*

Makes 4 servings

3 to 4 tablespoons organic or homemade mayonnaise (page 238)
2 to 3 garlic cloves
¼ cup olive oil
1 teaspoon fresh dill
1 teaspoon fresh parsley
1 teaspoon freshly squeezed lemon juice
1 to 2 drops of stevia (optional)

Spoon the mayonnaise into a small bowl, then use a garlic press to add the garlic to the bowl. Stir, then add the remaining ingredients. Store in the refrigerator for up to 4 days.

Caesar Salad Dressing

Makes up to 6 servings
1 tablespoon gluten-free Dijon mustard
Juice of ½ lemon
½ cup olive oil
1 teaspoon gluten-free Worcestershire sauce
7 anchovies, or 1 tablespoon anchovy paste
2 garlic cloves
Celtic sea salt
Purified water (optional)

Whisk the mustard and lemon juice together in a small bowl. Slowly drizzle in the olive oil until the mixture coats the backside of a spoon. Add the Worcestershire sauce. If you are using canned anchovies, drain and discard the anchovy oil. Using a garlic press, squeeze the garlic and anchovies into the mixture, or press the garlic and add the anchovy paste. You can also put half of the dressing into a blender to make it creamier, then add it back to the remaining half of the dressing. Add salt to taste, and add purified water by the tablespoon to thin the dressing, as needed. Store in a glass container in the refrigerator for up to 4 days.

Hearty Salads

Basic tips for making a great salad:

Always prewash your greens and veggies in grape seed extract (GSE) to eliminate any "critter" residue. To do this, fill a large stainless-steel salad bowl with about 8 cups of purified water. Add 8 drops of GSE. (Or, for smaller amounts of veggies, use 1 drop of GSE per cup of water.) Soak your veggies for anywhere from 30 seconds up to 1 minute.

Store washed lettuce in the refrigerator in a brown paper towel, which will help keep it crisp if you are washing your lettuce ahead of time, before you prepare your meals.

Baby Greens Side Salad

Makes 2 servings

6 cups baby greens

4 cherry tomatoes

2 teaspoons diced red onion

Combine all the ingredients in a medium-size bowl and toss with your favorite salad dressing. The salad will keep in the refrigerator for 24 hours.

Arugula Side Salad

Makes 2 servings

1 avocado (halve if using
   entire fruit)

5 cups arugula

½ cup sliced cucumber

2 teaspoons pine nuts (optional)

Slice the avocado into 1-inch segments, inside the peel. Scoop out the flesh, place it in a small bowl, and set aside. Combine the arugula, cucumber, and pine nuts, if using, in a medium-size bowl and toss gently. Add the avocado right before serving. Serve with your favorite salad dressing. The salad will keep in the refrigerator for 24 hours.

Kale Side Salad

Makes 2 servings

6 cups flat-leaf kale

Juice of ½ lemon

6 cherry tomatoes

3 tablespoons chopped red onion

6 to 8 walnuts, chopped

Celtic sea salt

Remove the kale leaves from the stems and discard the stems. Cut the kale into bite-size pieces and place in a medium-size bowl. Pour the lemon juice over the kale to soften it. Let sit for 1 minute before adding the cherry tomatoes, red onion, and walnuts. Add salt to taste. The salad will keep in the refrigerator for 24 hours.

Greek Side Salad

Makes 4 servings

4 to 6 cups chopped romaine lettuce	8 cherry tomatoes
8 kalamata olives	4 tablespoons pine nuts
	1 cucumber

Combine all the ingredients in a medium-size salad bowl and serve with your favorite salad dressing. The salad will keep in the refrigerator for 24 hours.

Nutty Greek Salad

Makes 6 servings

1 cucumber	12 kalamata olives, halved
1 cup cherry tomatoes	⅓ cup MCT Essential Salad Dressing (page 249)
2 to 3 tablespoons chopped red onion	½ cup pine nuts
8 to 12 cups romaine lettuce, chopped	½ cup organic hulled hemp seeds

Combine the cucumber, tomatoes, onion, lettuce, and olives in a large bowl. Toss with the MCT dressing. Add the pine nuts and hemp seeds, then serve immediately. The salad can be stored in the refrigerator for up to 2 days.

Greek Salad with Chicken

Makes 2 servings

1 tablespoon gluten-free Dijon mustard
Juice of 1 lemon
1 teaspoon olive oil
4 to 8 ounces diced chicken, or 6 to 8 organic chicken tenders
6 cups mixed greens, baby greens, or romaine lettuce
1 tomato, chopped
1 cucumber, chopped

½ red onion, chopped
Basil Salad Dressing (page 251)
2 tablespoons pine nuts

Whisk the mustard, lemon juice, and olive oil together in a shallow bowl. Marinate the chicken in the mixture for 30 minutes, then broil on LOW for 3 to 4 minutes on each side. Set aside. In a large bowl, toss the mixed greens, tomato, cucumber, and onion together with the basil salad dressing. Add the cooked chicken (warm or cold) and pine nuts and toss again before serving. The salad can be stored in the refrigerator for up to 24 hours.

Chinese Chicken Salad

Makes 2 to 4 servings
6 to 12 ounces diced chicken, or 6 to 12 organic chicken tenders
½ cup organic low-sodium chicken stock
21 Seasoning Salute (Trader Joe's) or other herbal seasoning
Dried thyme
Celtic sea salt
2 cups shredded napa or green cabbage
2 cups shredded red cabbage
1 Japanese cucumber, chopped
½ cup shredded carrot
Asian Marinade (page 246)
½ cup slivered almonds

Place the chicken, chicken stock, herbal seasoning, thyme, and salt to taste in a medium-size saucepan. Cook over low heat for 4 to 5 minutes, taking care not to overcook the chicken. When the chicken is tender, remove it from the heat and allow it to cool. Set aside.
In a large bowl, combine the veggies, then toss with the Asian marinade. Add the chicken and almonds. Toss the salad again and serve. The salad will keep in the refrigerator for up to 2 days.
Note: After the chicken is cooked, you can set aside the chicken broth and keep it as a soup base.

Curry Chicken Salad

Makes 2 servings

    1 tablespoon homemade mayonnaise (page 238)
    1 teaspoon MCT liquid coconut oil
    4 to 6 ounces cooked chicken, shredded or diced
    ½ cup chopped celery
    ¼ to ½ teaspoon curry powder
    A few golden raisins (optional)
    4 butter lettuce leaves, for serving

In a medium-size bowl, combine the mayonnaise and MCT oil, along with the cooked chicken, celery, and curry powder. Add the golden raisins, if desired. Scoop the mixture into the lettuce leaves and serve. The salad can be stored in the refrigerator for up to 2 days.

Chicken Caesar Salad

Makes 6 servings

    3 heads organic romaine lettuce
    1 to 2 cups chopped arugula
    ½ pound organic chicken tenders
    1 tablespoon gluten-free Dijon mustard
    Juice of 1 lemon
    2 tablespoons olive oil
    ½ cup almond meal
    ¼ cup coconut flour
    Celtic sea salt
    Freshly ground black pepper
    1 teaspoon Italian seasoning
    ½ teaspoon 21 Seasoning Salute (Trader Joe's) or other herbal seasoning
    Coconut oil, ghee (clarified butter), or palm oil, for sautéing
    ¼ teaspoon paprika
    2 Hard-Boiled Eggs (page 236), chopped
    Caesar Salad Dressing (page 252)
    Lemon wedges, for serving

Chop the washed lettuce and arugula into bite-size pieces, then place in a large salad bowl, cover with a damp paper towel, and place in the refrigerator.

In a separate bowl, toss the chicken tenders with the mustard and half of the lemon juice. Add the olive oil and toss again.

In a third bowl, combine the almond meal, coconut flour, salt, pepper, and Italian and herbal seasoning. Place the chicken tenders in the bowl and press them on all sides into the almond mixture.

Place the coconut oil in a medium-size saucepan and heat over medium heat. Add the coated chicken and sauté until crisp, 3 to 4 minutes per side. Alternatively, place the chicken in a medium-size baking pan and bake in a preheated 400°F oven for 14 to 15 minutes, or 7 minutes per side. Season the cooked chicken with the salt and paprika to taste.

Next, toss the prepared romaine lettuce and arugula, and add the chopped hard-boiled eggs and Caesar salad dressing to the bowl. Divide the salad among six individual plates and place three or four cooked chicken tenders on top of each salad. Drizzle additional salad dressing over the tenders. Place a lemon wedge on top of each salad and serve. The salad can be stored in the refrigerator for up to 24 hours.

Ceviche Salad

Makes 6 to 8 servings

4 cups purified water
1 cup freshly squeezed lemon juice (from 4 to 6 lemons)
1 pound freshwater scallops
1 pound freshwater shrimp
1 jalapeño pepper, seeded and diced
½ cup chopped green onions
2 organic tomatoes, seeded and diced
½ cup finely chopped fresh cilantro
1 to 2 avocados
Romaine lettuce or baby greens, for serving
Citrus Delight Dressing (page 250, optional), for serving

Place the water and 2 tablespoons of the lemon juice in a 6-quart pot. There should be just enough liquid to cover the seafood, once it is added to the pot. Bring the water to a gentle boil. Place the scallops and shrimp in the boiling water. Lower the heat to a simmer and cook the seafood for 2 to 3 minutes, just until the shrimp turn pink and the scallops are opaque. Do not overcook the seafood, or it may end up rubbery in texture. (It's best to slightly undercook it, as it will still continue to cook after you have removed it from the liquid.)

Place the seafood in a strainer and allow it to cool for about 10 minutes. Chop the shrimp and scallops into bite-size pieces and pour half of the remaining lemon juice over the seafood mixture.

Add the jalapeño, green onions, tomatoes, and cilantro to the seafood and toss. Chop the avocado flesh into medium-size chunks and add them to the seafood mixture. Add any remaining lemon juice. Chill and serve over the romaine lettuce, with the lemon dressing (see note). Can be stored in the refrigerator for up to 24 hours.

Alternatively, you can also toss the lettuce with Cilantro Dressing or MCT Dressing (pages 250 and 249) and then top your shrimp salad with it.

Seared Toasted Sesame Salmon Salad

Makes 6 servings

2 cups steamed green beans
1 cup water-based artichoke hearts
1 cucumber, sliced
12 kalamata olives
8 to 12 cups baby greens or arugula
1 cup cherry tomatoes

2 tablespoons organic capers
½ to 1 cup black sesame seeds
6 (3- to 4-ounce) salmon steaks
½ cup Asian Marinade (page 246)
Coconut oil, for pan
⅓ cup Citrus Delight Dressing (page 250), or to taste

Julienne the steamed green beans or slice into bite-size pieces, then set aside. Slice the artichoke hearts and cucumber into bite-size pieces and set aside. Slice the olives in half and set aside.

Place the greens in a large salad bowl, then add the artichoke hearts, cucumber, and olives and toss. Arrange the salad on individual plates. Arrange the green beans, tomatoes, and capers around each salad. Set aside.

Place the sesame seeds in a medium-size dry skillet and slightly toast over medium heat for a minute or two. Set the toasted seeds aside on a dinner plate.

Coat the salmon in the Asian marinade, leaving it in the marinade for 5 minutes per side. Remove the salmon from the marinade and firmly press
it into the toasted sesame seeds, ensuring that both sides of the salmon
are coated with seeds.

Sear the salmon in coconut oil in a 9-inch saucepan over medium heat or on
a flat griddle for 4 minutes per side. Place the seared salmon on top of
the salad. Drizzle the salmon and green beans with Asian dressing or the
citrus salad dressing and serve immediately. The salad can be stored in
the refrigerator for 24 hours.

Salmon Salad with Avocado

Makes 2 servings

4 to 6 ounces cooked fresh or canned salmon (If canned,
  use wild-caught salmon packed in water.)
6 cups spinach, washed, stems removed, cut into bite-size pieces
1 tablespoon chopped fresh parsley or dill
1 large tomato, cut into bite-size pieces
1 celery stalk, chopped into bite-size pieces
½ cucumber, chopped into bite-size pieces
¼ cup diced red onion
1 to 2 tablespoons olive oil, plus 1 teaspoon for pan
2 to 3 tablespoons freshly squeezed lemon juice
½ avocado, chopped into bite-size pieces
1 cup organic portobello mushrooms
2 tablespoons Asian Marinade (page 246) or Citrus Delight Dressing
  (page 250)

Place the salmon in a large bowl and mash into small chunks. Add the spinach, parsley, tomato, celery, cucumber, and half of the red onion and
toss gently. Add the olive oil and lemon juice and mix well. Fold the
chopped avocado into the salad mixture. Set aside.

Place the remaining teaspoon of olive oil in a 6-inch pan, and quickly sauté
the remaining red onion and the mushrooms over medium heat for
about 2 minutes, until soft. Add the mushroom mixture to the spinach
salad, toss with salad dressing, and serve. The salad can be stored in the
refrigerator for up to 24 hours.

Sautéed Scallops Seafood Salad

Makes 4 servings

½ cup organic low-sodium chicken stock
½ cup freshly squeezed lemon juice
3 garlic cloves, pressed
8 to 14 freshwater scallops
Fresh parsley sprigs
6 to 8 cups baby greens
1 cup steamed and sliced green beans
2 to 4 tablespoons Citrus Delight Dressing (page 250)
2 green onions, chopped
1 avocado, cut into bite-size pieces

Combine the chicken stock and lemon juice with the garlic in a 6- to 8-inch skillet. Heat the mixture over medium heat for about a minute, then drop in the scallops and cook them until they are opaque, about 4 minutes, taking care not to overcook them. Add the parsley and set aside.

In a large bowl, combine the baby greens, green beans, and zesty lemon dressing and toss. Top the salad with the scallops, green onion, and avocado and serve. The salad can be stored in the refrigerator for up to 2 days.

Filling Soups

The following soups are delicious, healthy, filling, and mineral- and nutrient-rich. They are also very soothing and satisfying to the body. They are an especially great meal option for those with compromised digestion, as soft, cooked foods are easier on the digestive tract. Most can be consumed as a stand-alone meal, but they also pair well with any side salad. The vegetable soups go well with any meat entrée.

Miso Broth with Mushrooms
Vegetable Soup
Vegetable Medley Soup
Creamy Broccoli/Cauliflower Soup
Chicken Vegetable Soup
Hearty Beef Soup
Seafood and Coconut Milk Soup with Cilantro and Chives

Miso Broth with Mushrooms

Makes 4 servings

1 bunch green onions or leeks

2 tablespoons chopped fresh cilantro leaves, stalks reserved

3 thin slices fresh ginger, peeled

2 star anise

1 small dried red chile

5 cups organic low-sodium vegetable or chicken stock

1 cup chopped portobello mushrooms

1 cup chopped bok choy or other Asian greens

4 tablespoons red miso paste

2 to 3 teaspoons tamari sauce or coconut amino acids

1 fresh chile, seeded and shredded, for garnish (optional)

Cut the coarse green tops off the green onions, reserving the green and white parts, then slice the tops finely on the diagonal. Place the tops in a large pot, along with the cilantro stalks, ginger, star anise, dried chile and vegetable stock.

Heat the mixture to a boil over medium heat, then lower the heat and simmer for about 10 minutes. Strain the vegetables out of the broth, return the broth to the pot, and reheat until simmering. Then, chop the onions into bite-size pieces and add the green pieces to the broth, along with the chopped mushrooms and bok choy. Set the white onion pieces aside. Cook the broth for 4 minutes.

In a small bowl, combine the miso with a little broth from the pot to make a paste, then stir the mixture into the pot. Add the tamari sauce.

Chop the white parts of the green onions. Stir most of the cilantro leaves into the soup, along with the white onion pieces. Cook for 1 minute, then ladle the soup into warmed serving bowls. Sprinkle the remaining cilantro and shredded fresh chile, if using, on top of the soup and serve. The soup is best when consumed immediately.

Vegetable Soup

The following recipe is vegetable-based, although you can also add chicken if you would like some extra protein in the dish.

Makes 6 servings
6 cups organic low-sodium chicken or vegetable stock
1 onion, chopped
1 cup celery, diced
1 garlic clove, pressed
1 cup cauliflower, cut into small pieces
2 cups shredded cabbage
½ cup fresh parsley, large stems removed and discarded, chopped
1 teaspoon dried oregano

In a large pot, combine the chicken stock, onion, celery, and garlic. Cook over medium heat until the vegetables are tender, about 5 minutes. Add the cauliflower and cabbage and simmer for 3 to 5 minutes. Add the herbs and serve. The soup can be stored in the refrigerator for 2 days or frozen.

Vegetable Medley Soup

Makes 4 servings
6 cups organic low-sodium chicken or vegetable stock
1 bay leaf
1 cup diced onion
1 cup diced leek
1 organic tomato, chopped
2 carrots, diced
1 cup diced Swiss chard
2 cups diced zucchini
1 cup diced celery
¼ teaspoon cayenne pepper
Celtic sea salt

Place the chicken stock in a large soup pot and bring to a boil. Add the bay leaf, onion, leek, tomato, and carrots. Lower the heat, simmer for about 15 minutes, then add the remaining ingredients, including salt to taste. Simmer until the zucchini and Swiss chard are tender, about 5 minutes or less. Taste and adjust the seasonings.

Creamy Broccoli/Cauliflower Soup

Makes 6 servings

  4 to 6 cups organic low-sodium chicken stock
  5 cups chopped broccoli or cauliflower
  2 carrots, peeled and cubed
  1 cup chopped leek (white parts only)
  1 cup chopped yellow onion
  ½ cup unsweetened almond milk or organic cream (optional)
  1 teaspoon dried basil
  Pinch of cayenne pepper
  Celtic sea salt, or Spike seasoning

Pour the chicken stock into a large soup pot. Add the broccoli, carrots, leek, and onion and simmer over medium heat for 5 to 10 minutes, until all the vegetables are tender but not mushy. Remove from the heat and let cool for 10 minutes. Ladle the ingredients into a blender, 2 cups at a time, and blend until smooth. Alternatively, use an immersion blender to mix the ingredients in the soup pot.

Return the mixture to the soup pot and simmer for 3 minutes. Add the almond milk or cream to the soup if the mixture is too thick, and simmer for just long enough to heat the milk, about 1 minute. Add the basil, cayenne, and salt to taste. You can freeze this soup or store it in the refrigerator for up to 2 days.

Chicken Vegetable Soup

For the first part of this recipe, you will be making a broth. If you don't end up using all of it for the soup, you can keep some of it to drink later or use any leftovers to make a vegetable soup.

Makes 8 servings

  1 whole organic chicken, including the innards
  About 10 cups purified water
  1½ cups chopped yellow onion
  4 celery stalks (including leaves), chopped
  2 bay leaves

    12 green and red peppercorns
    2 zucchini, chopped
    1 cup green beans, cut into 1-inch pieces
    Celtic sea salt
    1 teaspoon dried marjoram
    Avocado, for garnish (optional)

In a large pot, submerge the chicken in the water. Bring the water to a boil, then lower the heat and simmer for about 15 minutes. Skim off any foam. Add the onion along with the celery stalks and leaves, bay leaves, and peppercorns. Simmer the chicken for about 30 minutes, or until it is fully cooked. Remove the chicken from the liquid, then strain out and discard the vegetables and set the broth aside. Bone and dice or shred the chicken into small pieces.

To make the vegetable portion of the soup, add the zucchini, green beans, and marjoram to 8 cups of the broth. You can top off with purified water if you don't have a full 8 cups of broth. Simmer over medium heat for 10 minutes. Cook until the vegetables are tender, about 5 minutes, adding salt to taste. Add the chicken pieces back to the pot. Top off each serving of soup with a slice of avocado, if using. The soup can be frozen or stored in the refrigerator for up to 3 days.

Note: If you are using vegetable soups or side dishes as your main entrée at mealtimes, we recommend adding 5 to 10 capsules of MAP (Master Amino Acid Pattern) to your meals.

Hearty Beef Soup

This hearty beef soup takes some time to create, but is well worth the time, effort, and attention because it's so tasty and nutritious.

Makes 12 servings
    2 pounds beef chuck roast
    ¼ cup coconut flour
    1 teaspoon paprika
    1 teaspoon coarsely ground black pepper
    2 teaspoons Celtic sea salt, or to taste
    2 tablespoons extra-virgin olive oil

2 tablespoons unsalted organic butter

1 cup diced white onion

3 to 4 garlic cloves, minced

1 cup high-quality red wine

32 ounces (4 cups) organic low-sodium beef stock

2 teaspoons gluten-free Worcestershire sauce

1 tablespoon Italian seasoning

1½ cups chopped celery (bite-size pieces)

1 cup chopped baby carrot (bite-size pieces)

1 cup chopped zucchini (bite-size pieces)

1 cup chopped green beans (bite-size pieces)

Fresh parsley, for garnish (optional)

Trim the hard fat and silver skin (the white/silvery-looking skin) from the beef and cut into 1- to 1½-inch cubes. Set aside. Place the coconut flour, paprika, pepper, and a teaspoon of the salt in a 1-gallon resealable plastic bag. Seal the bag and shake, to mix all the contents. Add the beef and shake the bag again until the beef is well coated. Set the beef and bag aside.

Warm the olive oil in a large Dutch oven or heavy-bottomed pot over medium-high heat. Hold your hand 6 inches above the pot, and once you feel warmth in your hand, add the butter to the pot. Once the butter is melted, carefully add half of the beef, one piece at a time, shaking off any excess coating. Brown the beef on all sides. Remove the beef and set it aside on a large plate. Cook the remaining beef until browned and place on the plate. (It will not yet be fully cooked, so do not taste at this point.)

Scrape up the browned bits of food residue at the bottom of the pan, so that they will dissolve and combine with the remainder of the soup's ingredients. Add the onion, garlic, and wine and cook until the onion is translucent. Add the beef stock, Worcestershire sauce, remaining salt, and Italian seasoning and stir to combine all the ingredients.

Return the beef to the pot, then cover and bring the mixture to a boil. Then, lower heat and allow the soup to simmer for 40 minutes, until the meat is tender.

Add the vegetables to the pot and stir. Cook for 10 minutes, covered, or until the vegetables are fork-tender. Add the parsley, if using. This soup can be stored in the refrigerator for 2 days or divided into portions and frozen.

Seafood and Coconut Milk Soup
with Cilantro and Chives

The long list of ingredients in this Thai-inspired recipe might mislead you into thinking that this soup is complicated to make. However, it is actually very easy to put together.

You can find the asterisked ingredients at your local health food store (e.g., Trader Joe's, Ralph's, or Whole Foods) or in the international foods section of your local supermarket. Firm white fish or chicken may be substituted for the shrimp.

Makes 8 servings

> 6 cups organic low-sodium fish* or chicken stock
> 5 thin slices fresh ginger, peeled
> 2 fresh lemongrass stalks,* cut into 1-inch pieces
> Zest of 1 lime, or 2 kaffir lime leaves*
> 1 bunch of chives, chopped
> ¼ cup chopped fresh cilantro
> 1 tablespoon coconut oil
> 4 shallots, chopped
> 1 (14-ounce) can light coconut milk*
> 2 to 3 tablespoons Thai fish sauce*
> 3 to 4 tablespoons Thai green curry paste*
> 1 pound large uncooked shrimp, peeled and deveined
> 1 pound calamari, prepared and cut into rings
> 2 to 4 tablespoons freshly squeezed lime juice
> Celtic sea salt
> Thai red chili paste* (optional)

Pour the fish stock into a large, heavy pot. Add the ginger, lemongrass, and about half of the lime zest. Then add half of the chives, along with the cilantro. Bring the mixture to a boil, then lower the heat, cover, and simmer gently for 20 minutes. Strain the stock and discard the herbs.

In a small or medium-size saucepan, heat the coconut oil over medium heat and cook the shallots for a few minutes, until they just begin to brown. Then stir the shallots into the broth.

Add the coconut milk, the remaining lime zest, and 2 tablespoons of the fish sauce. Heat gently until simmering, then lower the heat and cook for 5 to 10 minutes. Add the Thai green curry paste, shrimp, and calamari and cook for another 3 to 5 minutes. Add the lime juice and season with more fish sauce, salt, and/or Thai red chili paste, to taste. Garnish with the chives. This soup can be frozen or stored in the refrigerator for 2 days.

Side Dishes

All of the following side dishes pair well with many of the entrées in the Recipes, such as Garlic Lemon Dijon Chicken (page 274), Seared Toasted Sesame Salmon Salad (page 258), or Versatile Meat Loaf (page 277). To stay in ketosis, choose one of these side dishes to eat daily for lunch or dinner, along with your protein entrée. All of these dishes are tasty; anti-inflammatory; low-glycemic; and fiber-, vitamin-, and mineral-rich. They are also simple to make and require little prep time.

Steamed Artichokes
Steamed Cauliflower Delight
Fennel with Turmeric
Steamed Dill Carrots
Roasted Zucchini and Eggplant

Steamed Artichokes

The artichoke dip can be used with the steamed artichokes, as well as a sauce over fish or burgers.

Makes 6 servings

6 artichokes   Juice of ½ lemon

ARTICHOKE DIP:
  2 tablespoons olive oil
  3 to 4 garlic cloves, crushed
  ¾ cup fresh or organic mayonnaise (page 238)
  1 teaspoon dried or fresh dill
  ½ to 1 teaspoon coconut amino acids
  1 teaspoon gluten-free Worcestershire sauce
  1 tablespoon freshly squeezed lemon juice

Cut the ends off of the artichokes with a serrated or bread knife and slice the artichokes in half down the middle. Place the artichokes in a vegetable steamer. Squeeze the lemon juice over the top and steam for about 30 minutes, or until the leaves pull away easily. With a spoon, scoop out the spiny center of each artichoke and discard it, taking care to not remove the edible tender parts.

To make the dip, heat the olive oil in a small saucepan over medium heat, add the garlic, and sauté until it is soft, about 5 minutes. Let the mixture cool slightly, then transfer to a small bowl. Add the mayonnaise, then the remaining ingredients. The dip can be stored in the refrigerator for up to 3 days.

Steamed Cauliflower Delight

Makes 4 servings
1 whole organic cauliflower
1 tablespoon organic salted or unsalted butter or ghee
1 to 2 tablespoons almond meal
⅓ cup organic low-sodium chicken or vegetable stock
Sprinkle of 21 Seasoning Salute (Trader Joe's) or other herbal
    seasoning blend
Sprinkle of Italian seasoning
1 teaspoon nutritional yeast flakes (optional, to add cheesy flavor)
2 tablespoons Pine Nut Dip (page 242) or organic heavy cream

Remove the cauliflower core and leaves. Steam the cauliflower whole for 15 minutes in a vegetable steamer. While the cauliflower is steaming, melt the butter in a medium-size saucepan over medium heat. Stir the almond meal into the butter, to make a paste, or roux. Stir in the chicken stock and season to taste with 21 Seasoning Salute, Italian seasoning, and nutritional yeast, if using, then add the pine nut dip or cream.

Remove the cauliflower from the steamer and transfer to a plate. Drizzle the roux, or mixture from the pan over the steamed cauliflower. To slightly brown the top of the cauliflower, place it on the lower shelf of your broiler, about 6 inches from the heat, and broil for about 2 minutes. The dish is best consumed right away, while warm.

Fennel with Turmeric

Fennel is an underused vegetable; pair it with turmeric and you have a health-supportive side dish that tastes great with fish or chicken.

Makes about 2 servings
> 1 tablespoon coconut oil
> ½ teaspoon ground turmeric
> 1 fennel bulb, leaves removed, sliced in half, then lengthwise

Heat the coconut oil over medium heat in a medium-size saucepan. Add the turmeric and sauté quickly, so that the spice blends into the oil. Place the fennel in the pan and sauté until tender, about 5 minutes. The dish is best consumed right away, while warm.

Steamed Dill Carrots

In place of or in addition to carrots, you can lightly steam other vegetables, such as asparagus, green beans, cauliflower, or Brussels sprouts, or a combination, for this recipe.

Makes 4 servings
> 4 carrots, sliced into small pieces
> 1 teaspoon olive oil
> 1 teaspoon minced fresh ginger
> 1 teaspoon dried dill
> 1 drop of stevia (optional)

Steam the carrots in a vegetable steamer until you can just pierce them with a fork. Place the oil and ginger in a medium-size saucepan and sauté for 1 minute over low heat. Add the carrots, dill, and stevia, if using, and sauté until heated through. The dish is best consumed right away, while warm.

Roasted Zucchini and Eggplant

Makes 4 servings

3 Japanese eggplants
½ teaspoon Celtic sea salt
3 medium-size zucchini
3 tablespoons olive oil
2 tablespoons coconut amino acids
6 to 8 large romaine lettuce leaves
½ cup Creamy Curry Dip (page 244)

Rinse the eggplants, then slice in half lengthwise. Add a few sprinkles of the salt, and set them in a colander to drain off any excess liquid, about 5 minutes.

Quarter the zucchini lengthwise. Place the zucchini and eggplant in a large bowl and toss with the olive oil and coconut amino acids. Broil the zucchini and eggplants on LOW for about 3 minutes, then flip them over and broil for another 3 minutes on the other side.

Spread out the lettuce leaves on a large plate or platter. Remove the vegetables from the broiler and place them on top of the leaves. Drizzle with the creamy curry dip. The dish is best consumed right away.

Easy Entrées

In keeping with the ketogenic or other low-carbohydrate anticancer diet, all the following entrées should be paired with either a vegetable side dish, side salad, and/or a lettuce wrap. All the following dishes are low-glycemic and protein-rich, to help the body to maintain a stable blood sugar and fulfill its essential amino acid needs. Amino acids help the body rebuild itself, maintain muscle mass, and support immune function. For optimal digestion, consume only one type of protein per meal. If you choose an entrée that does not contain an animal protein, such as zucchini noodles, be sure to take some MAP capsules or Body Health amino acids (see Chapter 4) with your meal.

Zucchini Noodles
Baby Rack of Lamb
Filet Mignon
Dijon Dill Salmon
Tex-Mex Turkey Wraps
Herb Almond Crusted Chicken or Mahimahi
Garlic Lemon Dijon Chicken
Chili Beef Wraps
Ground Chicken or Turkey Patties (with Lettuce Wrap)
Versatile Meat Loaf
Garlic Herbed Shrimp

Zucchini Noodles

Vegetable "noodles" are easy to make and are so good for you! You can purchase a vegetable spiralizer or simply use a vegetable peeler to create your noodles.

Makes 3 to 4 servings
   4 medium-size zucchini
   4 cups purified water

Place the zucchini in the vise of a spiralizer and follow the manufacturer's instructions. If you are making the noodles by hand, use your vegetable peeler to create long strips. After all the zucchini has been sliced into thin strips, place the strips in a colander. Then, boil the water and pour the hot water over the zucchini strips, which will make the noodles warm and a bit soft, but still raw. (If you prefer, the zucchini can also be sautéed in a medium-size saucepan in a tablespoon of olive oil over medium heat for 2 to 4 minutes, for a more cooked dish.) Drain the zucchini. Mix with your favorite sauce and serve. It is best to consume this dish right away, while still warm.

Baby Rack of Lamb

Makes 2 servings

2 (3- to 4-ounce) lamb chops
¼ cup Lamb Marinade (page 245)

Soak the chops in the lamb marinade for 20 minutes or longer. Place the chops in a broiler pan and place in the oven 6 inches away from broiler. Broil for 3 minutes on each side and serve.

Filet Mignon

Makes 2 servings

2 (3.5- to 5-ounce) filet mignon steaks
4 tablespoons Asian Marinade (page 246)

Marinate the steaks in the Asian marinade for 10 minutes or longer. Place the filets on a broiler pan and place in the oven 6 inches away from the broiler. Broil for 3 to 4 minutes on each side and serve. The dish may be kept in the refrigerator for 2 to 3 days. To reheat, pour ¼ cup of chicken stock into a medium-size saucepan. Bring to a boil, lower the heat, then add the steaks. Cover and heat for 2 to 3 minutes.

Dijon Dill Salmon

Makes 2 servings

1 tablespoon gluten-free Dijon mustard	1 teaspoon dried dill
Juice of ½ lemon	3 tablespoons olive oil
4 garlic cloves	2 (4-ounce) wild salmon fillets
	Coconut or olive oil spray

Whisk the mustard, lemon juice, garlic, dill, and olive oil together in a shallow bowl, to make a marinade. Coat the salmon on both sides with the marinade and let sit for 10 minutes in a shallow baking dish.

Prepare an 8- to 9-inch baking dish by lightly coating it with coconut oil spray. Place the salmon in the prepared dish and place in the oven at least 6 to 8 inches away from the broiler. Broil for 4 minutes per side. It's best to slightly undercook the fish, which will help retain its moisture. The cooked salmon can be stored in the refrigerator for 2 days.

Tex-Mex Turkey Wraps

Makes 4 servings

2 to 4 tablespoons coconut or palm oil

½ to ¾ white onion

1½ cups chopped portobello mushrooms

1 pound ground turkey

½ jalapeño pepper, diced and seeded, or a pinch of cayenne pepper (optional)

½ teaspoon dried cumin

½ teaspoon paprika

1 teaspoon chipotle powder

Celtic sea salt

1 tablespoon Bragg Liquid Aminos

PER SERVING:

12 to 16 butter or romaine lettuce leaves (3 to 4 leaves per serving)

2 tablespoons Fresh Guacamole (page 240)

1 tablespoon Fresh Salsa (page 240)

In a small skillet over medium heat, heat 2 tablespoons of the coconut oil. Add the onion and sauté until it is slightly translucent, about 2 minutes. Add the mushrooms to the pan and cook until they are tender, 1 to 2 minutes. Remove the mushroom mixture from the pan and set aside in a small bowl.

Add the remaining 2 tablespoons of coconut oil to the skillet, and sauté the ground turkey over medium heat for about 10 minutes, breaking up the meat into small pieces as you cook it. Once it is browned, add the spices, salt, and liquid aminos to taste, and cook over low heat for another 5 minutes. Add the mushroom mixture, cover with a lid, and cook for an additional 5 minutes.

Wrap in the lettuce leaves or place over a bed of leaves on a plate. Top with guacamole and salsa and enjoy. Store in the refrigerator for up to 2 days.

Herb Almond Crusted Chicken or Mahimahi

Although this recipe calls for chicken or mahimahi, you can use any white fish or turkey cutlets.

Makes 2 servings

3 tablespoons coconut oil
1 heaping tablespoon gluten-free Dijon mustard
1 teaspoon olive oil
½ cup almond meal
1 teaspoon dried thyme
1 teaspoon dried rosemary
1 teaspoon 21 Seasoning Salute (Trader Joe's) or other herbal
    seasoning blend
1 teaspoon garlic powder
Celtic sea salt
2 (3- to 4-ounce) skinless chicken breasts or mahimahi fillets

Preheat the oven to 450°F. Coat the bottom of an 8- to 9-inch baking dish
    with the coconut oil. Set aside.
Whisk the mustard and olive oil together in a small bowl. In a separate bowl
    or plate, whisk together the almond meal, herbs, and salt to taste.
Coat the chicken in the mustard mixture, then the herbal mixture. Place the
    prepared baking dish in the preheated oven and leave it there until the
    oil is hot and bubbling. Place the herb-coated chicken in the hot dish
    and bake for 10 minutes, until the chicken is browned and moist. You
    can broil the chicken during the last minute of cooking to make it crisp,
    but take care to not overcook or burn the crust. The chicken or fish can
    be stored in the refrigerator for up to 2 days.

Garlic Lemon Dijon Chicken

Makes 2 servings

2 tablespoons gluten-free Dijon mustard
1 tablespoon olive oil
5 garlic cloves, crushed

3 tablespoons freshly squeezed lemon juice
1 teaspoon Italian seasoning
½ teaspoon paprika
1 teaspoon lemon zest
7 ounces chicken breast
Coconut oil, for pan

Whisk together all the ingredients, except the chicken and coconut oil, in a
medium-size bowl to make a marinade. Place the chicken breast in the
marinade, coating it completely on both sides.

Grease a 6- to 8-inch baking pan with coconut oil and add the chicken. Place
the chicken in the oven about 6 inches from broiler. Broil for 3 to
4 minutes on each side, taking care to not overcook. The chicken can
be stored in the refrigerator for up to 2 days.

Chili Beef Wraps

*These wraps are high in protein and flavor, but make a very light meal due to
the wraps, which are made of lettuce. Serve with fresh salsa and guacamole for a
healthy, delicious lunch or dinner.*

Makes 2 servings
2 tablespoons coconut oil
½ cup chopped onion
7 ounces organic ground beef
1 tablespoon tomato paste
2 tablespoons purified water
½ teaspoon dried dill
1 teaspoon garlic powder
1 teaspoon chili powder
½ to 1 teaspoon ground cumin
½ teaspoon paprika
6 to 8 large butter or romaine lettuce leaves (3 or 4 leaves per serving)
¼ cup Fresh Salsa (page 240)
A dollop of Fresh Guacamole (page 240)

Melt the coconut oil in a medium-size skillet over medium heat. When the
   oil is hot, add the onion and cook for about 5 minutes, until the onion
   is translucent. Add the ground beef and continue to cook over medium
   heat, breaking up the beef into taco-size pieces as you cook it.

Add the tomato paste, then the water. Stir, then add the dill, garlic, chili,
   cumin, and paprika. Simmer the mixture over low heat for about 20
   minutes.

Serve the beef warm inside butter leaf lettuce wraps or over romaine lettuce,
   with the salsa and guacamole. The dish can be stored in the refrigerator
   for up to 2 days.

Ground Chicken or Turkey Patties (with Lettuce Wrap)

*You can substitute ground organic beef for the chicken or turkey in this recipe.
You can also use any of the mayonnaise sauce recipes in the Dips section (pages
238–239) as a garnish for the burgers.*

Makes 2 servings
   1 teaspoon garlic powder
   ¼ to ⅓ cup Bragg Liquid Aminos
   6 to 8 ounces ground chicken or turkey
   ½ jalapeño pepper, diced (optional)
   Coconut oil spray, for pan
   1 tablespoon coconut oil
   1 cup chopped red onion
   6 to 8 butter lettuce or Swiss chard leaves (3 or 4 leaves per patty)
   Sliced avocado or cucumber, for serving (optional)
   Celtic sea salt (optional)

Mix the garlic powder and half of the liquid aminos together in a medium-size bowl until well blended. Add the chicken and mix thoroughly.

Form the chicken into two equal-size patties. Set aside.

In a separate bowl, mix together the remaining liquid aminos and the jalapeño, and allow the mixture to sit in the bowl for 10 minutes. This will
   help the amino acids absorb the pepper flavor.

Marinate the patties in the amino acid mixture for about 2 minutes on each
   side. Then, prepare a medium-size skillet by spraying with coconut oil

into it. Place the patties in the skillet (reserving any leftover marinade) and cook over medium heat for 3 to 4 minutes on each side, or to your desired doneness.

While the patties are cooking, in a small saucepan over medium heat, heat the tablespoon of coconut oil along with any remaining marinade from the burgers, and sauté the onion until it becomes translucent, about 5 minutes. Remove from the heat.

After the burgers are finished cooking, cut them into three or four pieces, then wrap each piece in a lettuce leaf and top with the onion mixture. Serve with sliced avocado or cucumber, and salt to taste, if desired. The burgers can be stored in the refrigerator for up to 2 days.

Versatile Meat Loaf

You can substitute beef, chicken, or turkey for the ground meat in this recipe. Serve over a bed of steamed kale or lettuce.

Makes 4 servings
> Coconut or olive oil, for pan
> 1½ pounds ground beef
> ½ cup minced onion
> ½ cup minced fresh parsley
> 1 teaspoon Italian seasoning
> 1 tablespoon almond meal
> 1 large egg
> 2 teaspoons Bragg Liquid Aminos
> Pinch of cayenne pepper
> 2 to 3 tablespoons ketchup

Preheat the oven to 350°F. Grease a 6- to 8-inch loaf pan with coconut oil.

In a medium-size bowl, thoroughly combine the ground beef and all the other ingredients, except for the ketchup. Form the meat into a loaf and place in the prepared pan. Spread the ketchup over top of the loaf. Bake the meat loaf for 15 to 30 minutes. Store in the refrigerator for up to 2 days.

Garlic Herbed Shrimp

Makes 3 to 4 servings

    8 to 12 ounces raw shrimp
    1 to 2 tablespoons coconut oil or ghee
    6 garlic cloves, chopped or pressed
    2 tablespoons chopped fresh cilantro or parsley
    1 cup diced cucumber
    Celtic sea salt
    1 tablespoon sesame seeds, for garnish (optional)
    4 cups shredded raw cabbage, for serving
    Creamy Garlic Dressing (page 251), if serving cold

Clean, devein, and remove the shells from the shrimp. If the shrimp are large, cut them down the middle. Set aside.

Heat the coconut oil in a medium-size saucepan over medium heat. Add the garlic and sauté for about 1 minute. Do not overbrown the garlic. Add the shrimp and cook for 2 to 3 minutes, until the shrimp are pink on all sides.

Add the cilantro and cucumber and season to taste with Celtic sea salt. Sprinkle with the sesame seeds, if using. Serve over the cabbage. If you are using raw cabbage, consider adding the creamy garlic dressing to make a tasty salad. The cooked shrimp can be stored in the refrigerator for up to 2 days.

Simple Snacks and Desserts

The following snacks and desserts were created to satisfy your sweet tooth and curb any sugar or fat cravings, while also enabling you to fulfill the requirements of a nutritious low-carb diet. They are satisfying, filling, and easy to make. Enjoy them, but eat sparingly as a treat, not as a substitute for your main meals.

Crunchy Seed Snack Mix
Sprouted Nuts
Toasted Nuts
Cheesy Cashew Kale Chips

Deviled Eggs
Raw Low-Carbohydrate Chocolate Squares
Cinnamon Chia Pudding

Crunchy Seed Snack Mix

Makes 6 to 8 servings

1 cup sunflower seeds
1 cup raw pumpkin seeds
2 cups purified water
¼ cup coconut amino acids

Soak the seeds in the water for 6 hours, then drain and pat them dry. Place them on a cookie sheet and sprinkle the coconut amino acids over them to coat.

Place the cookie sheet in a cold oven and set the oven to the lowest temperature, or 150° to 170°F, and oven-dry for 5 hours, or until the seeds are crisp. Store in an airtight container in the refrigerator, where they will keep for several weeks.

Sprouted Nuts

Sprouted nuts are very healthy for the body because soaking nuts draws the healthful enzymes out of them and makes them easy for the body to digest. They are also simple to make.

Makes about 4 servings

1 cup almonds or other nuts (walnuts, cashews, Brazil nuts, etc.)
2 cups purified water

Soak the nuts in the water for 6 hours, then drain and pat dry. Sprouted nuts don't keep for long; they get moldy fairly quickly. So, store in the fridge for no longer than 48 hours. The nuts can also be frozen.

Toasted Nuts

Makes about 4 servings
1 cup soaked raw almonds or walnuts
Garlic powder (optional)
Ground cumin (optional)

Place the nuts on a cookie sheet, and coat with garlic powder and/or cumin.
Place the cookie sheet nuts in a cold oven and set the oven to the lowest
temperature, or 150° to 180°F, and oven-dry for about 3½ hours. Store
in a mason jar for up to several weeks. The nuts can also be frozen.
Tip: For sweet nuts, add ground cinnamon and a bit of stevia, instead of the
garlic or cumin.

Cheesy Cashew Kale Chips

*For this recipe, you'll want to completely dry the washed kale pieces so as to pro-
duce kale chips with a maximum amount of crunch. Consider even washing your
kale the day before you prepare this recipe and leave the pieces to dry overnight in
a paper towel in the refrigerator, to soak up any excess moisture.*

Makes 4 servings
2 medium-size bunches flat leaf or curly kale (4 cups leaves once
    bite-size)

CASHEW CHEESE SAUCE
1 cup cashews (soaked overnight for at least 6 hours)
1 medium-size red bell pepper, seeded and roughly chopped
Juice of ½ lemon
½ cup nutritional yeast
½ teaspoon garlic powder
½ teaspoon Celtic sea salt, or to taste
Pinch of cayenne pepper, dried dill, or onion powder (optional)
Chipotle chile powder (optional)

Begin with unwashed kale. Trim off the toughest part of the kale stems, then cut or tear the leaves into bite-size pieces. Fill a large bowl with water and add the kale pieces. Swish the kale around so that any debris floats to the top. Drain and dry completely in a salad spinner or with towels. Once the kale is dry, place the dried pieces in a large bowl with enough room to mix the kale with the cashew cheese sauce.

Prepare the cashew cheese sauce: Combine the soaked cashews, bell pepper, lemon juice, nutritional yeast, garlic powder, sea salt, and cayenne, dill, or onion powder, if using, in a high-powered blender or food processor. A high-powered blender, such as a Vitamix, is ideal for this. Blend the ingredients together until smooth.

Mix the cheese sauce with the dried kale, using your hands to massage the sauce into the kale. It doesn't matter if the coating is uneven or there are big globs of cashew cheese on the kale.

Preheat the oven to 200°F and spread the kale pieces over parchment-lined baking sheets. Bake for 45 minutes, or until crunchy. Or, if you have a dehydrator, follow the manufacturer's instructions to dehydrate the kale, for an even crispier chip. To add additional kick to this recipe, add a pinch of cayenne or chipotle chile powder to the chips. The kale can be stored in a resealable plastic bag for up to a week.

Deviled Eggs

Makes 4 servings

> 4 Hard-Boiled Eggs (page 236)
> 1 tablespoon organic or homemade mayonnaise (page 238)
> ¼ teaspoon gluten-free Dijon mustard
> Pinch of paprika
> Pinch of dried dill
> Celtic sea salt

Slice the hard-boiled eggs in half. Remove the yolks and place in a small bowl. Set the egg whites aside. Mash the egg yolks with a fork and combine with the mayonnaise, mustard, paprika, dill, and salt to taste. Spoon the yolk mixture back into the center of the egg whites. The eggs will keep in the refrigerator for 24 hours.

Raw Low-Carbohydrate Chocolate Squares

Makes about 20 small squares

¾ cup coconut oil
1 cup almond meal
2 large scoops low-carb, plant-based chocolate protein powder,
    such as PlantFusion
2 tablespoons raw cacao powder
½ cup coarsely chopped walnuts
Ground cinnamon
Pinch of Celtic sea salt
3 drops of stevia, or to taste

Line a 6-inch baking pan with waxed paper and set aside. Place the coconut
    oil in a 1-quart saucepan and heat over medium heat for 2 minutes,
    until it becomes a liquid. Remove the pan from the heat and add all the
    other ingredients one at a time, including cinnamon to taste, stirring
    the mixture with a spoon until it resembles a thick brownie mix.
Pour the mixture into the lined pan, spreading it out evenly until it is about
    ¼ inch thick across the pan. Place the pan in the freezer and freeze for
    10 minutes. Remove from the freezer and slice the chocolate bars into
    1-inch squares. Place them back in the freezer and freeze for another
    20 minutes, then remove and enjoy one piece at a time with love! Store
    the remaining bars in the freezer in a glass container.

Cinnamon Chia Pudding

Makes 2 servings

1 to 2 cups Brazil nut, almond, or coconut milk
1 teaspoon pure vanilla extract
⅓ cup chia seeds
1 to 2 tablespoons stevia, to taste
Pinch of ground cinnamon
Pinch of Celtic sea salt (optional)

Mix all the ingredients together in a bowl until smooth and creamy, using a large spoon. Let the mixture sit for 10 minutes, then stir again. Add more almond milk to reach your desired consistency. Then, allow it to sit for at least another 30 minutes, or for optimum taste and nutritional benefits, store overnight in the refrigerator.

FOR a more protein-rich meal, add ¼ cup of hemp seeds along with 2 to 3 tablespoons of raw sunflower seeds (soaked for 8 to 12 hours) and/or 1 to 2 tablespoons of shredded unsweetened coconut to the basic chia mixture. You can also add ½ cup of kefir, for a creamier consistency, and/or some raw berries, such as raspberries or blueberries, for added flavor. For a mousselike variation, whip up ½ cup of organic heavy whipping cream and stir into the chia pudding.

Metric Conversions

The recipes in this book have not been tested with metric measurements, so some variations might occur.

Remember that the weight of dry ingredients varies according to the volume or density factor: 1 cup of flour weighs far less than 1 cup of sugar, and 1 tablespoon doesn't necessarily hold 3 teaspoons.

General Formula for Metric Conversion

Ounces to grams	multiply ounces by 28.35
Grams to ounces	multiply grams by 0.035
Pounds to grams	multiply pounds by 453.5
Pounds to kilograms	multiply pounds by 0.45
Cups to liters	multiply cups by 0.24
Fahrenheit to Celsius	subtract 32 from Fahrenheit temperature, multiply by 5, divide by 9
Celsius to Fahrenheit	multiply Celsius temperature by 9, divide by 5, add 32

Weight (Mass) Measurements

1 ounce = 30 grams
2 ounces = 55 grams
3 ounces = 85 grams
4 ounces = ¼ pound = 125 grams
8 ounces = ½ pound = 240 grams
12 ounces = ¾ pound = 375 grams
16 ounces = 1 pound = 454 grams

Volume (Liquid) Measurements

1 teaspoon = ⅙ fluid ounce = 5 milliliters
1 tablespoon = ½ fluid ounce = 15 milliliters
2 tablespoons = 1 fluid ounce = 30 milliliters
¼ cup = 2 fluid ounces = 60 milliliters
⅓ cup = 2⅔ fluid ounces = 79 milliliters
½ cup = 4 fluid ounces = 118 milliliters
1 cup or ½ pint = 8 fluid ounces = 250 milliliters
2 cups or 1 pint = 16 fluid ounces = 500 milliliters
4 cups or 1 quart = 32 fluid ounces = 1,000 milliliters
1 gallon = 4 liters

Volume (Dry) Measurements

¼ teaspoon = 1 milliliter
½ teaspoon = 2 milliliters
¾ teaspoon = 4 milliliters
1 teaspoon = 5 milliliters
1 tablespoon = 15 milliliters
¼ cup = 59 milliliters
⅓ cup = 79 milliliters
½ cup = 118 milliliters
⅔ cup = 158 milliliters
¾ cup = 177 milliliters
1 cup = 225 milliliters
4 cups or 1 quart = 1 liter
½ gallon = 2 liters
1 gallon = 4 liters

Linear Measurements

½ in = 1½ cm
1 inch = 2½ cm
6 inches = 15 cm
8 inches = 20 cm
10 inches = 25 cm
12 inches = 30 cm
20 inches = 50 cm

Oven Temperature Equivalents, Fahrenheit (F) and Celsius (C)

100°F = 38°C	250°F = 120°C	350°F = 180°C	450°F = 230°C
200°F = 95°C	300°F = 150°C	400°F = 205°C	

Resources and Further Reading

CANCER CENTER FOR HEALING WEBSITES

Cancer Center for Healing: www.CancerCenterforHealing.com

Perfectly Healthy (Dr. Connealy's supplements): www.PerfectlyHealthy.com

Newport Natural Health (Dr. Connealy's newsletter): www.NewportNatural
Health.com

PRACTITIONER REFERRAL WEBSITES

Academy for Comprehensive Integrative Medicine: www.acimconnect.com

American College for Advancement in Medicine: www.acam.org

Huggins Applied Healing: www.HugginsAppliedHealing.com

International Academy of Oral Medicine and Toxicology: http://iaomt.org/

International Organization of Integrative Cancer Physicians: www.ioicp.com

Chapter 2: How to Detect Cancer Before It Wreaks Havoc

TESTING LABORATORIES

BioMeridian, BioScan MSA: http://biomeridian.com. To find a BioMeridian practitioner, see Alternatives for Healing holistic medicine directory:
http://www.alternativesforhealing.com/. Go to "Find a practitioner"
tab on website.

Cancer Profile: American Metabolic Laboratories and Metabolic Research,
Inc., www.AmericanMetabolicLaboratories.net

C-reactive protein and other routine blood tests: Any lab, such as Quest
Diagnostics or LabCorp. (You can also order these tests at DirectLabs
.com or LabTestsOnline.org.)

LSA Limbic Stress Assessment System (LSA): ZYTO Corporation, www
.Zyto.com
ONCOblot: ONCOblot Labs, www.ONCOblotlabs.com
RGCC: Research Genetic Cancer Center (RGCC), http://rgcc-genlab.com
Thermography:
International Academy of Clinical Thermology, http://www.iact-org. Click
on "links" to find a thermography practitioner.
Pink Image Breast Thermography: www.Mypinkimage.com

Chapter 3: Groundbreaking Cancer Treatments

TREATMENTS AND ASSOCIATED ORGANIZATIONS
Autohemotherapy and Ultraviolet Blood Irradiation:
Issels Immuno-Oncology: http://issels.com. Click on "Treatments."
UVL (RX) Therapeutics: www.uvlrx.com
Goleic: FirstiMMUNE: http://immunocentre.eu. Click on "Treatments" link.
Hyperbaric Oxygen Therapy:
www.HBOT.com
International Hyperbarics Association: http://www.ihausa.org
IPT:
www.IPTQ.com
www.IPTforcancer.com
Best Answer for Cancer foundation: www.bestanswerforcancer.org
IV Curcumin: "Curcumin: Can It Really Prevent Cancer?" Cancer Center
for Healing, http://www.newportnaturalhealth.com. Type "curcumin"
into website search box.
IV Vitamin C:
Cancer Tutor: www.CancerTutor.com
Dr. Whitaker: America's Most Trusted Wellness Doctor, http://www
.drwhitaker.com. Type article name: "IV vitamin C kills cancer cells"
into website search box.
Live Cell Therapy: Peptides Store: www.peptidesstore.com
PEMF: www.PEMF.com, www.PEMF.us
Supportive Oligonucleotide Technique (SOT): Cancer Center for Healing, http://www.cancercenterforhealing.com. Type "SOT" into website
search box.

Chapter 4: Let Food Be Your Medicine

PRODUCTS
Amino Acid Meal Supplements:
Master Amino Acid Pattern (MAP) Supplements: www.masteraminoacid-
pattern.com
Dosage: See Chapter 12.
Perfect Amino by Body Health: http://bodyhealth.com. Click on "products"
and then "Perfect Amino."
Dosage: Same as MAP.
Clean Organic Meat Products: US Wellness Meats: www.USWellnessMeats
.com
Drinking Water Filters:
Berkey filters: www.Berkeyfilters.com
Chanson alkaline water filters: www.chansonalkalinewater.com
pHenomenal water: www.phenomenolwater.com
pH Prescription Water, LLC: www.phprescription.com
purative.com
Plant Protein Powders:
NutraFusion Nutritionals: PlantFusion
Nutiva Hemp Protein: http://nutiva.com/hemp/
Sunwarrior Warrior Blend Raw Vegan Protein: www.SunWarrior.com/store
Super Protein in the Buff by Boku Superfoods: www.Bokusuperfood.com

RECOMMENDED READING
"Five Things You Should Know About GMOs." Environmental Working
Group (August 21, 2012). Accessed March 1, 2015, http://www.ewg
.org/research/five-things-you-should-know-about-gmos.
Johansson, L. *The Protein Revolution.* Information4Life, 2014.
Moore, J. *Keto Clarity: Your Definitive Guide to the Benefits of a Low-Carb,
High-Fat Diet.* Victory Belt Publishing, August 5, 2014.
Seyfried, T. *Cancer as a Metabolic Disease: On the Origin, Prevention and
Treatment of Cancer.* Wiley, 2012.

Chapter 5: Remove Toxins to Boost Your Health

HOME AND BODY PRODUCTS/TREATMENTS
Air Purifiers:
Austin Air: www.austinair.com.
Bee Propolis Air Purifiers: Be Healthy Farms: www.beHealthyFarms.com
Biological Dentistry:
International Academy of Biological Dentistry and Medicine: http://iabdm
    .org/
International Academy of Oral Medicine and Toxicology: iaomt.org
Building Biologists: International Institute for Building Biology and Ecol-
    ogy: http://hbelc.org
Chi Machine: Chi Machine International: www.chimachine4u.com.
Coffee Enema Preparation: Center for New Medicine: http://cfinmedicine
    .com. Input "coffee enema protocol" into website search box.
EMF Protection Products:
Earthing and Grounding Products: www.Earthing.com
EMF Safety Superstore: www.lessemf.com
Graham-Stetzer filters: www.stetzerelectric.com
Sauna Companies:
Frisby Portable Dry Sauna: www.Sears.com and other retail outlets
Health Mate: www.healthmatesauna.com

SUPPLEMENTS
Chlorella: Sun Chlorella: www.Sunchlorellausa.com
    Dosage: 5 to 30 tablets daily, according to your doctor's instructions
Zeolite: NutraMedix zeolite: www.NutraMedix.com
    Dosage: 2 or more capsules daily
Energique Chelatique: http://www.energiqueherbal.com/
    Dosage: Take according to product instructions.

TESTING COMPANIES
Diagnos-Techs: www.Diagnostechs.com
Genova: https:www.gdx.net

PRACTITIONER REFERRAL WEBSITES
Academy for Comprehensive Integrative Medicine: www.acimconnect.com
       American College for Advancement in Medicine: www.acam.org
International Organization of Integrative Cancer Physicians: www.ioicp.com

RECOMMENDED READING

Becker, R. *Cross Currents: The Perils of Electropollution*, (New York: Penguin, 1990).

Benson, J. "Seven Amazing Health Benefits of Coffee Enemas," Natural News.com, December 21, 2012. Accessed March 1, 2015, http://www.naturalnews.com/038429_health_benefits_coffee_enema_detox.html.

"Cancer," Pesticide Action Network North America. Accessed January 8, 2015, http://www.panna.org/your-health/cancer.

Crofton, K. *A Wellness Guide for the Digital Age: With Safer-tech Solutions for All Things Wired & Wireless—For Brains Worth Saving*, 3rd ed. Global Wellbeing Books, 2013.

Chapter 6: Harness the Power of Supplements

TESTING

Estrogen Testing: Estronex Profile: www.estronex.com

Nutrient Testing:

NutrEval, Genova Diagnostics: https://www.gdx.net. Type "NutrEval nutritional test" into website search box.

SpectraCell Laboratories: www.SpectraCell.com

FERMENTED FOODS

Rejuvenative Foods: www.rejuvenative.com

CANCER TREATMENT SUPPLEMENTS

Artemisinin: Allergy Research Group: http://www.allergyresearchgroup.com/artemisinin

Dosage: 2 capsules twice daily

CoQ10: CoQ-Zyme 100 Plus: www.BioticsResearch.com. (Any brand is okay.)

Dosage: 300 to 400 mg daily

Curcumin:

Newport Natural Health Curcumin EX Plus: https://store.newportnaturalhealth.com.

Thorne Research Labs, Meriva 500: https://www.thorne.com.

Dosage: 500 mg, 3x/day

Essiac Tea: Essiac Canada International: www.EssiacProducts.com.

Dosage: Take as directed on the product label.

Green Tea Extract: Any brand at your local health food store.

    Dosage: Take as directed on the product label, or 2 capsules, 2x/day.

Indole-3-carbinol: Any brand at your local health food store.

    Dosage: 1 capsule, 2x/day

Melatonin:

Melatonin Sleep Solution: https://store.newportnaturalhealth.com/

Nature Made melatonin: www.naturemade.com/Melatonin.

    Dosage: 1 to 3 mg before bedtime to improve sleep. For cancer treatment, take 10 to 20 mg before bedtime, or according to your doctor's instructions.

Mushrooms:

Combination Mushroom Product: Host Defense My Community Capsules: www.fungiperfecti.com

Dosage: Take according to product instructions

Dr. Chi's Cordyceps Extract and Reishi Spore Extract (for both cancer prevention and treatment): Available at many online retailers.

Dosage: Take according to product instructions for cancer prevention purposes; take according to your doctor's instructions for cancer treatment purposes.

Mushroom Science: Maitake and chaga (for both cancer prevention and treatment)

    Available at: www.mushroomscience.com. Type "maitake" and/or "chaga" into website search box.

    Dosage: Take according to product instructions for cancer prevention purposes; take according to your doctor's instructions for cancer treatment purposes.

Quercetin:

Biotics Research, Bio-FCTS: www.BioticsResearch.com

    Dosage: 2 capsules, 2x/day

Thorne Research, Quercetin Phytosome: https://www.thorne.com. Type "quercetin" into website search box.

    Dosage: Take according to your doctor's instructions.

DIGESTIVE SUPPLEMENTS

Digestive Enzymes: Maxi-Health Enzymax: http://www.maxihealth.com. Type "Enzymax" into website search box.

Hydrochloric Acid: Any brand at your local health food store.

Probiotics: Theralac: http://www.theralac.com/

    Dosage: Take according to product instructions.

Maxi-Health Floramax: http://www.maxihealth.com. Input "Floramax" into
   website search box.
   Dosage: Take according to product instructions.

FOUR CORE SUPPLEMENTS

Pancreatic Enzymes:

Nutrizyme, by American Nutraceuticals: http://www.perfectlyhealthy.com.
   Type "Nutrizyme" into website search box.
   Dosage: 3 capsules, 2x/day for cancer prevention. Up to 10 capsules,
   3x/day for cancer treatment or per your doctor's recommendations.

P-A-L Plus, Get Healthy Again: http://www.gethealthyagain.com. Type
   "PAL enzymes" into website search box.
   Dosage: 3 capsules, 2x/day for cancer prevention. Up to 10 capsules,
   3x/day for cancer treatment or per your doctor's recommendations.

Wobenzyme Professional Strength: Can be found at a variety of online retailers.
   Dosage: 3 capsules, 2x/day for cancer prevention. Up to 10 capsules,
   3x/day for cancer treatment or per your doctor's recommendations.

Vitalzym, by World Nutrition Incorporated: www.worldnutrition.net.
   Dosage: 3 capsules, 2x/day for cancer prevention. Up to 10 capsules,
   3x/day for cancer treatment or per your doctor's recommendations.

Parent Essential Oils (PEOs) (alpha-linoleic and linoleic EFAs):

Yes Parent Essential Oils: http://www.yes-supplements.com/
   Dosage: 4 or more capsules daily

Udo's Oil 3–6–9 brand: Can be found at many online retailers.
   Dosage: Take according to product label instructions or your doctor's
   recommendations.

Vitamin C:

Allergy Research Group, Micro Liposomal C: http://www.allergyresearch
   group.com/. Type "Micro Liposomal C" into website search box.
   Dosage: 1 teaspoon, 2 to 3 times daily

American Nutriceuticals, Vitality C: www.888vitality.com. Type "Vitality C"
   into website search box.
   Dosage: 1,000 to 12,000 mg daily, per your doctor's recommendations.

Vitamin D:

Bio-D-Mulsion Forte, Biotics Research: www.BioticsResearch.com. Type
   "Bio-D Mulsion Forte" into website search box.
   Dosage: 5,000 to 15,000 IU daily

D-10,000, Thorne Research: https//Thorne.com. Type "D-10,000" into
   website search box.
   Dosage: 1 capsule daily

RECOMMENDED READING
Pauling, L., and Ewan Cameron. *Cancer and Vitamin C.* (Warner Books, 1981).

Chapters 7 and 8: Get Moving to Get Well;
Reduce Stress and Reclaim Your Life

AROMATHERAPY PRACTITIONERS
National Association of Holistic Therapy: www.naha.org

PRODUCTS
Bath Salts: Aura Cacia: www.AuraCacia.com
Chi Machine: Chi Machine International: www.chimachine4u.com
Essential Oil:
DoTerra: http://www.doterra.com/
Young Living: www.youngliving.com/
Meditation/Relaxation CDs:
HeartMath: www.HeartMath.org
Holosync: www.centerpointe.com
Jon Kabat-Zinn guided meditation CD series: http://www.mindfulnesscds
    .com.

MORE INFORMATION AND PRACTITIONER REFERRALS
Recall Healing: Renaud, G. Recall Healing: http: www.recallhealing.com.
    Click on "Resources" tab on website and then "Practitioners" to find a
    practitioner.
Qigong and Tai Chi: Alternatives for Healing: http://www.alternativesfor
    healing.com. Click on "Find a practitioner" tab on website.
Oncology Massage: Society for Oncology Massage: http://s4om.org/.
The Destination Method (TDM): www.teloscenter.com.

RECOMMENDED READING
Prinster, T. *Yoga for Cancer: A Guide to Managing Side Effects, Boosting Immunity, and Improving Recovery for Cancer Survivors.* Healing Arts Press, 2014.
Talbott, S. *The Cortisol Connection: Why Stress Makes You Fat and What You Can Do About It,* 2nd ed. (Hunter House, 2007).

Chapter 9: Strengthen Your Immune System with Sleep

AUDIO SLEEP CDS AND OTHER SLEEP TECHNOLOGY
Heart Math Institute Products:
Coherence Coach CD: store.heartmath.org
emWave2 With Solution for Better Sleep: store.heartmath.org
Inner Balance iOS 30 Pin Sensor & Better Sleep Solution: store.heartmath
.org
Solving Sleeplessness audio program: store.heartmath.org
Holosync audio CDs: www.centerpointe.com

SLEEP APNEA TESTING
American Academy of Sleep Medicine's Sleep Education site: www.sleep
education.com

SLEEP SUPPLEMENTS
GABA: Metabolic Maintenance: http://www.metabolicmaintenance.com.
Type "GABA" into website search box.
Dosage: 500 mg, 1 to 3/night
L-tryptophan: Thorne Research: https://www.thorne.com. Click on "amino
acids" under the "Products" tab on website.
Dosage: 500 to 1,500 mg before bedtime.
Melatonin: Melatonin Sleep Solution Kit, Newport Natural Health Store:
www.Store.NewportNaturalHealth.com. Type "melatonin" in product
search box on website.
Dosage: 1 to 3 mg before bedtime
5-HTP: Thorne Research: https://www.thorne.com. Click on "amino acids"
under the "Products" tab.
Dosage: 100 to 300 mg before bedtime
4Sleep [contains 5-HTP, GABA and glutamine], Perfectly Healthy: www
.PerfectlyHealthy.com.
Smart Pill IQ Maximizer: www.PerfectlyHealthy.com

HORMONE AND NEUROTRANSMITTER TESTING
Diagnos-Techs: www.DiagnosTechs.com
Meridian Valley Lab: www.MeridianValleyLab.com
Sabre Sciences: www.SabreSciences.com

RECOMMENDED READING
Kharrazian, D. *Why Isn't My Brain Working?* Elephant Press, 2013.

Chapter 10: Putting Together Your Support Team

RESOURCES
To Find a Cancer Support Group: Yahoo groups, https://www.yahoogroups
.com. Input "cancer" or "cancer support" into website search box.
To Find an Integrative Doctor or Other Practitioner: See the organizations
list at the beginning of the Resources.
To Raise Financial Support for Treatments: GoFundMe.com.

Chapter 11: Creating an Anticancer Living Environment

PERSONAL CARE AND HOUSEHOLD PRODUCTS
Air Purifiers:
Austin Air: www.AustinAir.com
Bee Propolis purifiers: Bee Healthy Farms: www.BeeHealthyFarms.com
Clean, Organic Meat and Seafood:
US Wellness Meats: www.grasslandbeef.com
Vital Choice Seafood: www.VitalChoice.com
EMF Protection Products:
EMF Safety Superstore: www.lessemf.com
Graham-Stetzer filters: www.stetzerelectric.com
Mold Testing:
Environmental Relative Moldiness Index (ERMI): www.mycometrics.com
Natural, Nontoxic Carpeting:
EarthWeave: www.EarthWeave.com
Nature's Carpet: www.NaturesCarpet.com
Personal Care and Household Cleaning Products:
Aubrey Organics: www.Aubrey-Organics.com
Dr. Bronner's: www.drbronner.com
Earth Easy: www.EarthEasy.com (Recipes to make your own cleaning products)
EarthWeave: www.earthweave.com
Eminence: www.EminenceOrganics.com
Green Shield: www.GreenShieldOrganic.com
Mrs. Meyer's: www.mrsmeyers.com

Nature's Carpet: www.naturescarpet.com
Osmosis: www.OsmosisSkinCare.com
Seventh Generation: www.SeventhGeneration.com
Weleda: www.Weleda.com.
Zum Zum: www.IndigoWild.com
Water Filtration Products and Systems:
Aquasana: www.aquasana.com
Berkey water filers: www.berkeyfilters.com
pH Prescription Water www.phprescription.com
pHenomenal Water: www.pHenomenalwater.com
purative.com

PRACTITIONER REFERRAL WEBSITES
American College for Advancement in Medicine (ACAM): acam.org.
    (See also the beginning of the References List.)

RECOMMENDED READING
Cowden, L. and Connie Strasheim, *Create a Toxin-Free Body & Home Start-ing Today*. ACIM Press, 2014, 87–98.
Environmental Working Group website: www.ewg.org (for studies on toxins
    in the home).
Shoemaker, R. *Mold Warriors*. Baltimore: Gateway Press, Inc., 2005.

Chapter 12: The 14-Day Anticancer Wellness Plan

PRODUCTS AND RESOURCES
Blood Ketone Meters: Abbott's Precision Xtra meter: Available at most phar-macies and box store retailers, such as Wal-Mart.
Food Calculators:
My Fitness Pal: www.myfitnesspal.com
My Food Diary: www.myfooddiary.com

RECOMMENDED READING
Moore, J. *Keto Clarity: Your Definitive Guide to the Benefits of a Low-Carb, High-Fat Diet*. Victory Belt Publishing, 2014.

The Recipes: Dishes for Repairing and Restoring the Body
Plant and Whey Protein Powders:
PlantFusion (NutraFusion Nutritionals): Available at many online retailers.
Nutiva Hemp Protein: www.Nutiva.com. Also available at many online retailers and health food stores.
Reservage Organics Grass-Fed Whey Protein: www.Reservage.com. Available at many online retailers.
Sunwarrior Warrior Blend Raw Vegan Protein: www.SunWarrior.com. Also available at many online retailers and health food stores.
Super Protein in the Buff (Boku Superfoods): www.Bokusuperfood.com.
TerasWhey Organic Whey Protein: www.Teraswhey.com. Also available at many online retailers and health food stores.

Notes

CHAPTER 1: CANCER: WHAT IT IS, WHAT CAUSES IT, AND HOW TO FIGHT IT

1. G. Morgan, R. Ward, and M. Barton, "The Contribution of Cytotoxic Chemotherapy to 5-Year Survival in Adult Malignancies," *Clinical Oncology* (*Royal College of Radiologists*) 16, no. 8 (December 2004): 549–60.

2. "Family Cancer Syndromes," American Cancer Society, last modified June 25, 2014, http://www.cancer.org/cancer/cancercauses/geneticsandcancer/heredity-and-cancer.

3. http://www.ncbi.nlm.nih.gov/pmc/articles/PMC3046088/; Thomas R. Cox and Janine T. Erler, "Remodeling and Homeostasis of the Extracellular Matrix: Implications for Fibrotic Diseases and Cancer," *Diseases and Model Mechanisms* 4, no. 2 (March 2011): 165–78.

4. Christoph Augner, Gerhard W. Hacker, and Ilse Jekel, "Geopathic Stress Zones: Short-Term Effects on Work Performance and Well-Being," *Journal of Alternative and Complementary Medicine* 16, no. 6 (2010): 657–61.

5. Eunice Virtanen, Birgitta Söder, Leif C. Andersson, Jukka H. Meurman, and Per-Östen Söder, "History of Dental Infections Associates with Cancer in Periodontally Healthy Subjects: A 24-Year Follow-Up Study from Sweden," *Journal of Cancer* 5, no. 2 (2014): 79–85, doi: 10.7150/jca.7402.

6. D. J. Shah, R. K. Sachs, and D. J. Wilson. "Radiation-Induced Cancer: A Modern View," *British Journal of Radiology* 85, no. 1020 (2012): e1166–e1173, doi: 10.12 59/bjr/25026140.

"Do X-rays and Gamma Rays Cause Cancer?" American Cancer Society, last modified February 24, 2015, http://www.cancer.org/cancer/cancercauses/geneticsandcancer /heredity-and-cancer, http://www.cancer.org/cancer/cancercauses/radiationexposureand cancer/xraysgammaraysandcancerrisk/x-rays-gamma-rays-and-cancer-risk-do -xrays-and-gamma-rays-cause-cancer. There have been cohort studies that follow a population of people who have been exposed to large amounts of ionizing radiation. For example, one study assessed the prevalence of cancer in the population of the Japanese atomic bomb survivors of World War II. The study found that increased levels of exposure led to increased cancer prevalence. Atomic bomb survivors had higher incidences of leukemia, multiple myeloma, thyroid cancer, bladder cancer, breast cancer, lung cancer, ovarian cancer, colon cancer, esophagus cancer, stomach cancer, liver cancer, lymphoma, and skin cancer. The information above is also confirmed by the American Cancer Society.

7. http://www.cancer.gov/about-cancer/coping/feelings/stress-fact-sheet.

8. "The Cancer Cascade," American Medical Research, LLC (October 2004).

9. Otto Warburg, "The Prime Cause and Prevention of Cancer," Nobel-Laureates, Lake Constance, Germany, June 30, 1966.

10. A. M. Port, M. R. Ruth, and N. W. Istfan, "Fructose Consumption and Cancer: Is There a Connection?" *Current Opinion in Diabetes, Endocrinology, and Obesity* 19, no. 5 (2012): 367–74, doi: 10.1097/MED.0b013e328357f0cb.

11. "The Cancer Cascade."

12. "Overweight and Obesity Statistics," National Institute of Diabetes and Digestive and Kidney Disease, last modified October2012, http://www.niddk.nih.gov/health-information/health-statistics/Pages/overweight-obesity-statistics.aspx#top.

CHAPTER 2: HOW TO DETECT CANCER
BEFORE IT WREAKS HAVOC

1. Emil Schandl, interview by Connie Strasheim, Alternative Cancer Research Institute, December 2014.

2. "Common Cancer Types," National Cancer Institute, accessed November 20, 2014, http://www.cancer.gov/cancertopics/types/commoncancers.

3. C. J. Wright, "Screening Mammography and Public Health Policy: The Need for Perspective," *Lancet* 346, no. 8966 (July 1995): 29–32, http://www.thelancet.com/journals/lancet/article/PIIS0140–6736(95)92655–0/abstract.

4. J. D. Brooks, W. E. Ward, J. E. Lewis, J. Hilditch, L. Nickell, E. Wong, and L. U. Thompson, "Supplementation with Flaxseed Alters Estrogen Metabolism in Postmenopausal Women to a Greater Extent Than Does Supplementation with an Equal Amount of Soy," *American Journal of Clinical Nutrition* 79, no. 2 (2004): 318–25, http://www.ncbi.nlm.nih.gov/pubmed/14749240.

5. R. Ablin, "The Great Prostate Mistake," *New York Times*, March 9, 2010.

6. http://sperlingprostatecenter.com/mri-vs-color-doppler-in-detecting-prostate-cancer/.

CHAPTER 3: GROUNDBREAKING CANCER TREATMENTS

1. A. Beisecker, M. R. Cook, J. Ashworth, J. Hayes, M. Brecheisen, L. Helmig, S. Hyland, and D. Selenke, "Side Effects of Adjuvant Chemotherapy: Perceptions of Node-Negative Breast Cancer Patients," *Psycho-oncology* 6, no. 2 (1997): 85–93, http://www.ncbi.nlm.nih.gov/pubmed/9205966.

2. L. Shyamala, H. C. Girish, and Sanjay Murgod, "Risk of Tumor Cell Seeding Through Biopsy and Aspiration Cytology," *Journal of International Society of Preventive and Community Dentistry* 4, no. 1 (2014): 5–11, doi: 10.4103/2231–0762.129446.

3. "Chemotherapy damages the genes inside the nucleus of cells. Some drugs damage cells at the point of splitting. Some damage the cells while they are making copies of all their genes before they split. Cells that are at rest, for instance most normal cells, are much less likely to be damaged by chemotherapy. You may have a combination of different chemotherapy drugs. The combination will include chemotherapy drugs that damage cells at different stages in the process of cell division. So, with more than one type of drug, there is more chance of killing more cells. The fact that chemotherapy drugs kill dividing cells helps to explain why chemotherapy causes side effects. It affects healthy body tissues where the cells are constantly growing and dividing. The skin, bone marrow, hair follicles and lining of the digestive system (gut) are examples of cells that are constantly growing and dividing." "How Chemotherapy Works," Cancer Research UK, last modified December 13, 2014, http://www.cancerresearchuk.org/about -cancer/cancers-in-general/treatment/chemotherapy/about/how-chemotherapy-works.

4. "Cancer Treatment and Survivorship Facts and Figures 2014–2015," American Cancer Society, http://www.cancer.org/acs/groups/content/@research/documents /document/acspc-042801.pdf.

5. "Cancer Facts and Figures," American Cancer Society (2014), accessed April 21, 2015, http://www.cancer.org/acs/groups/content/@research/documents/webcontent /acspc-042151.pdf.

6. R. Webster Kehr, "Insulin Potentiation Therapy (IPT)," Independent Cancer Research Foundation, Inc., last updated May 31, 2016, https://www.cancertutor.com /ipt/. According to Steven G. Ayre, MD, in the book *Treating Cancer with Insulin Potentiating Therapy*, IPT can be used more frequently and has less negative side effects than chemotherapy. Insulin increases the delivery efficiency of chemotherapy to cancer cells; however, since insulin and chemotherapy are paired together in this treatment, a lower dose of chemotherapy is administered. A lower dose of administered chemotherapy results in fewer negative side effects.

7. Y. Jiang, Y. Pan, P. R. Rhea, L. Tan, M. Gagea, L. Cohen, S. M. Fischer, and P. Yang, "A Sucrose-Enriched Diet Promotes Tumorigenesis in Mammary Gland in Part Through the 12-Lipoxygenase Pathway," *Cancer Research*, January 1, 2016.

8. A. Alabaster, B. Vonderhaar, and S. Shafie, "Metabolic Modification by Insulin Enhances Methotrexate Cytotoxicity in MCF-7 Human Breast Cancer Cells," *European Journal of Cancer & Clinical Oncology* 17, no. 11 (1981): 1223–28.

9. Linus Pauling and E. Cameron, *Cancer and Vitamin C: A Discussion of the Nature, Causes, Prevention, and Treatment of Cancer with Special Reference to the Value of Vitamin C*, Updated and Expanded (Philadelphia: Camino Books, 1993).

10. C. G. Moertel, interview on *Health Report*, ABC National Radio, August 7, 1989, cited in Evelleen Richards, *Vitamin C and Cancer: Medicine or Politics?* (New York: St. Martin's Press, 1991).

11. American College of Physicians (ACP), "How Vitamin C Is Administered Affects How Much Reaches the Bloodstream and May Affect the Results of Studies of Its Potential Effect on Cancer," *Annals of Internal Medicine, Summaries for Patients* (April 6, 2004), accessed December 3, 2014, http://www.annals.org/cgi/content/full /140/7/533.

12. SOT is still in the process of clinical trials in the United States. Center for New Medicine is one of the pioneer facilities that is trying to begin clinical trials for this treatment. Further information about SOT can be found on the RGCC website, http://www.rgcc-group.com.

13. Subash C. Gupta, Sridevi Patchva, and Bharat B. Aggarwal, "Therapeutic Roles of Curcumin: Lessons Learned from Clinical Trials," *American Association of Pharmaceutical Scientists Journal* 15, no. 1 (2012): 195–218, doi: 10.1208/s12248-012-9432-8.

14. "Paul Niehans." Wikipedia, accessed April 2, 2015, http://en.wikipedia.org/wiki/Paul_Niehans.

15. Vladimir Khackelevich Khavinson, Clinical Study of Vladonix, International Association of Gerontology and Geriatrics (IAGG), accessed from PeptidesStore.com, http://www.peptidesstore.com/pages/clinical-study-of-vladonix.

16. Richard Nuccitelli et al., "Nanosecond Pulsed Electric Fields Cause Melanomas to Self-Destruct. PEMF and Skin Cancer," *Biochemical and Biophysical Research Communications* 343, no. 2 (May 5, 2006): 351–60.

CHAPTER 4: LET FOOD BE YOUR MEDICINE

1. Thomas Seyfried, *Cancer as a Metabolic Disease: On the Origin, Prevention and Treatment of Cancer* (Hoboken, NJ: Wiley, 2012).

2. Otto Heinrich Warburg, Wikipedia, accessed March 1, 2015, http://en.wikipedia.org/wiki/Otto_Heinrich_Warburg.

3. Joseph Mercola, "The Benefits of a Ketogenic Diet and Its Role in Cancer Treatment," Mercola.com, June 16, 2013, accessed March 1, 2015, http://articles.mercola.com/sites/articles/archive/2013/06/16/ketogenic-diet-benefits.aspx.

4. Dongil Choi, Jae Hoon Lim, Dong-Chull Choi, Seung Woon Paik, Sun-Hee Kim, and Sun Huh, "Toxocariasis and Ingestion of Raw Cow Liver in Patients with Eosinophilia," *Korean Journal of Parasitology* 46, no. 3 (2008): 139–43, doi: 10.3347/kjp.2008.46.3.139. There have been incidents of toxocariasis due to ingestion of raw cow liver, but research on this topic is sparse and the results were only able to conclude positive risk for patients with eosinophilia. For cancer patients and patients with suppressed immune systems, Dr. Connealy recommends taking HCL to aid digestion of raw liver.

5. F. Wu et al., "Global Risk Assessment of aflatoxins in Maize and Peanuts: Are Regulatory Standards Adequately Protective?" Toxicological Sciences (September 2013); Clay McNight, "Fungal Contamination of Peanuts," Livestrong.com, last modified September 9, 2015, http://www.livestrong.com/article/553348-fungal-contamination-of-peanuts/.

6. J. Sethi, M. Yadav, K. Dahiy., S. Sood, V. Singh, and S. B. Bhattacharya. "Antioxidant Effect of Triticum aestivium (Wheat Grass) in High-Fat Diet-Induced Oxidative Stress in Rabbits," *Methods and Findings in Experimental Clinical Pharmacology* 32, no. 4 (2010): 233, doi: 10.1358/mf.2010.32.4.1423889.

7. C. Lee et al., "Fasting Cycles Retard Growth of Tumors and Sensitize a Range of Cancer Cell Types to Chemotherapy," *Science Translational Medicine* (February 8, 2012).

8. R. Klement, "Calories, Carbohydrates, and Cancer Therapy with Radiation: Exploiting the Five R's Through Dietary Manipulation," *Cancer and Metastasis Reviews* (January 17, 2014), accessed January 5, 2015, http://link.springer.com/article/10.1007%2Fs10555–014–9495–3/fulltext.html.

9. "Five Things You Should Know About GMOs," Environmental Working Group (August 21, 2012), accessed March 1, 2015, http://www.ewg.org/research/five-things-you-should-know-about-gmos.

10. G. E. Seralini et al., "Long Term Toxicity of a Roundup Herbicide and a Roundup-Tolerant Genetically Modified Maize," *Food and Chemical Toxicology* 50, no. 11 (November 2012): 4221–31, doi: 10.1016/j.fct.2012.08.005.

CHAPTER 5: REMOVE TOXINS TO BOOST YOUR HEALTH

1. P. Gao et al., "Health Impact of Bioaccessible Metal in Lip Cosmetics to Female College Students and Career Women, Northeast of China," *Environmental Pollution* (November 25, 2014), doi: 10.1016/j.envpol.2014.11.006.

2. "Cancer," Pesticide Action Network North America, accessed January 8, 2015, http://www.panna.org/your-health/cancer.

3. Ibid.

4. Robert Becker, *Cross Currents: The Perils of Electropollution* (New York: Penguin, 1990).

5. Jonathan Benson, "Seven Amazing Health Benefits of Coffee Enemas," *Natural News,* December 21, 2012, accessed March 1, 2015, http://www.naturalnews.com/038429_health_benefits_coffee_enema_detox.html.

6. Ibid.

7. "Detox Tips 7: What Is Infrared?" DrEddyClinic.com, accessed January 10, 2015, http://www.dreddyclinic.com/detox_tips_7.htm.

8. W. Blumer and Elmer Cranton, "Ninety Percent Reduction in Cancer Mortality after EDTA Chelation Therapy with EDTA," *Journal of Advancement in Medicine* 2, no. 1/2 (Spring/Summer 1989), accessed January 9, 2015, http://gordonresearch.com/inner.cfm?itemCategory=46873&priorId=46695.

CHAPTER 6: HARNESS THE POWER OF SUPPLEMENTS

1. "High-Dose Vitamin C (PDQ®)-Patient Version," National Cancer Institute, last modified December 11, 2015, http://www.cancer.gov/about-cancer/treatment/cam/patient/vitamin-c-pdq.

2. Linus Pauling and Ewan Cameron, *Cancer and Vitamin C* (Philadelphia: Warner Books, 1981).

3. National Institutes of Health Dietary Supplement Label Database, http://www
.dsld.nlm.nih.gov/dsld/dailyvalue.jsp, accessed June 24, 2016; https://www.consumer
lab.com/RDAs/#VitaminC, accessed June 24, 2016.

4. George Ebers, "Vitamin D Found to Influence over 200 Genes, Highlighting
Links to Disease," Wellcome Trust Centre for Human Genetics, University of Oxford
(2010), http://www.well.ox.ac.uk/aug-10-vitamin-d-influences-over-200-genes.

5. Brian Peskin, "Why We Now Recommend Cardio Crusaders Parent Essential
Oils Instead of Fish Oil," Cardio Crusaders, accessed January 19, 2015, http://www
.brianpeskin.com/BP.com/about/CardioCrusaders.pdf.

6. John Beard, *The Enzyme Treatment of Cancer and Its Scientific Basis* (New York:
New Spring Press, 2009).

7. Oregon State University, "Gut Microbes Closely Linked to Proper Immune
Function, Other Health Issues," *Science Daily* (September 16, 2013), accessed January
19, 2015, http://www.sciencedaily.com/releases/2013/09/130916122214.htm.

8. "Quercetin Is a Multi-Faceted Cancer Fighter," Quercetin.com, accessed January 10, 2015, http://www.quercetin.com/cancer/quercetin-is-a-multi-faceted-cancer
-fighter.

9. E. Mills et al., "Melatonin in the Treatment of Cancer: A Systematic Review of
Randomized Controlled Trials and Meta-analysis," *Journal of Pineal Research* 39, no. 4
(November 2005): 360–66.

10. "The Healing Power of Artemisinin," accessed January 10, 2015, http://www
.artemisinin101.com/Artemisinin-Anti-Cancer.html.

11. "Garlic and Cancer Prevention," National Cancer Institute, January 2008,
accessed January 10, 2015, http://www.cancer.gov/cancertopics/factsheet/Prevention
/garlic-and-cancer-prevention.

12. R. T. Kodali and G. D. Eslick, "Meta-analysis: Does Garlic Intake Reduce Risk
of Gastric Cancer?" *Nutrition and Cancer* 67, no. 1 (January 2015): 1–11, doi: 10.1080
/01635581.2015.967873.

CHAPTER 7: GET MOVING TO GET WELL

1. "Physical Activity and Cancer," National Cancer Institute, accessed February
10, 2015, http://www.cancer.gov/cancertopics/factsheet/prevention/physicalactivity;
Cheryl L. Rock, "Nutrition and Physical Activity Guidelines for Cancer Survivors,"
CA: A Cancer Journal for Clinicians, University of California, San Diego, La Jolla, April
26, 2012.

2. "Physical Activity and Cancer."

3. M. L. Slattery, "Physical Activity and Colorectal Cancer," *Sports Medicine* 34,
no. 4 (2004): 239–52.

4. I. Lee and Y. Oguma, "Physical Activity," in *Cancer Epidemiology and Prevention*, 3rd ed. (New York: Oxford University Press, 2006).

5. IARC Handbooks of Cancer Prevention, *Weight Control and Physical Activity*,
vol. 6 (2002); R. Ballard-Barbash et al., "Obesity and Body Composition," in *Cancer*

Epidemiology and Prevention, 3rd ed., ed. David Schottenfeld and Joseph F. Fraumeri Jr. (New York: Oxford University Press, 2006); Lee and Oguma, "Physical Activity."

6. M. D. Holmes et al., "Physical Activity and Survival After Breast Cancer Diagnosis," *Journal of the American Medical Association* 293, no. 20 (2005): 2479–86.

7. M. Aleixo et al., "Physical Exercise Prior and During Treatment Reduces Sub-Chronic Doxorubicin-Induced Mitochondrial Toxicity and Oxidative Stress," *Mitochondrion* (November 7, 2014): 22–33, doi: 10.1016/j.mito.2014.10.008.

8. Y. M. Na et al., "Exercise Therapy Effect on Natural Killer Cell Cytotoxic Activity in Stomach Cancer Patients After Curative Surgery," *Archives of Physical and Medical Rehabilitation* 81 (2000): 777–79; C. Peters et al., "Influence of a Moderate Exercise Training on Natural Killer Cytotoxicity and Personality Traits in Cancer Patients," *Anticancer Research* 144 (1994): 11033–36.

9. Hye-Ryun Hong, "Effect of Walking Exercise on Abdominal Fat, Insulin Resistance and Serum Cytokines in Obese Women," *Journal of Exercise Nutrition & Biochemistry* 18, no. 3 (September 2014): 277–285, doi: 10.5717/jenb.2014.18.3.277 [Epub September 10, 2014].

10. Stephen J. Genuis et al., "Blood, Urine, and Sweat (BUS) Study: Monitoring and Elimination of Bioaccumulated Toxic Elements," *Archives of Environmental Contamination and Toxicology* 62, no. 2 (August 2011): 344–57, PMID: 21057782 [Epub November 6, 2010].

11. Margaret E Sears et al., "Arsenic, Cadmium, Lead, and Mercury in Sweat: A Systematic Review," *Journal of Environmental and Public Health* (2012): 184745, PMID: 22505948 [Epub February 22, 2012].

12. Sarah Tilyou, "Exercise May Reduce Risk of Certain Cancers," Oncology Times (August 15, 1987); R. E. Frisch et al., "Lower Prevalence of Non-Reproductive System Cancers Among Former College Athletes," *Medicine and Science in Sports and Exercise* 21, no. 3 (1989): 250–53.

13. A. J. Romain et al., "Effects of Exercise Training on Blood Rheology: A Meta-Analysis," *Clinical Hemorheology and Microcirculation* 49, no. 1–4 (2011): 199–205, doi: 10.3233/CH-2011-1469.

CHAPTER 8: REDUCE STRESS AND RECLAIM YOUR LIFE

1. "Psychological Stress and Cancer," National Cancer Institute, accessed January 25, 2015, http://www.cancer.gov/cancertopics/factsheet/Risk/stress.

2. Ibid.

3. Razalli Saleh Mohd, "Chronic and Acute Stress, Including Surgery and Social Disruptions, Appear to Promote Tumor Growth," *Malaysian Journal of Medical Sciences* 15, no. 4 (October 2008): 9–18.

4. Michael J. Mackenzie et al., "Affect and Mindfulness as Predictors of Change in Mood Disturbance, Stress Symptoms, and Quality of Life in a Community-Based Yoga Program for Cancer Survivors," *Evidence-Based Complementary and Alternative Medicine* (2013), accessed January 25, 2015, http://dx.doi.org/10.1155/2013/419496.

5. Chris Streeter et al., "Effects of Yoga Versus Walking on Mood, Anxiety, and Brain GABA Levels," *Journal of Alternative and Complementary Medicine* 16, no. 11 (November 2010): 1145–52, doi: 10.1089/acm.2010.0007.

6. L. Cohen et al., "Psychological Adjustment and Sleep Quality in a Randomized Trial of the Effects of a Tibetan Yoga Intervention in Patients with Lymphoma," *Cancer* 100, no. 10 (May 15, 2004): 2253–60.

7. T. Prinster, "Benefit #8 Yoga Helps Manage Fear and Anxiety," *Y4C.com Blog*, accessed February 1, 2015, http://y4c.com/category/benefits/.

8. D. Martarelli et al., "Diaphragmatic Breathing Reduces Postprandial Oxidative Stress," *Journal of Alternative and Complementary Medicine* 17, no. 7 (July 2011): 623–28, doi: 10.1089/acm.2010.0666 [Epub June 20, 2011].

9. Ginny Fraser, "Qigong—The Power to Heal," CANCERactive, accessed on February 10, 2015, http://www.canceractive.com/cancer-active-page-link.aspx?n=1438.

10. Ibid.; Luke Chan, "World's Largest Medicineless Hospital," *ChiLel*, accessed February 10, 2015, http://www.chilel.com/WhatIsChilelQigong/hospital.htm.

11. Richard Walters, "Chinese Medicine and Cancer," in *Options: The Alternative Cancer Therapy Book* (Garden City, NY: Avery Publishing, 1993).

12. Y. Zeng et al. "Health Benefits of Qigong or Tai Chi for Cancer Patients: A Systematic Review and Meta-analyses," *Complementary Therapies in Medicine* 221, no. 1 (February 2014): 173–86.

13. M. Hernandez-Reif et al., "Natural Killer Cells and Lymphocytes Increase in Women with Breast Cancer Following Massage Therapy," *International Journal of Neuroscience* 115, no. 4 (April 2005): 495–510.

14. B. Siegel, letter to the editor "Clarifications," *Massage Therapy Journal* 35, no. 2 (1996): 12.

15. "Aromatherapy." University of Maryland Medical Center, accessed January 25, 2015, http://umm.edu/health/medical/altmed/treatment/aromatherapy#ixzz3QcC4vBDl.

16. "Aromatherapy (Essential Oils Therapy): Topic Overview," WebMD, accessed February 10, 2015, http://www.webmd.com/balance/stress-management/tc/aromatherapy-essential-oils-therapy-topic-overview.

17. Michelle Schrader, "The Experience of Recall Healing: An Interpretative Phenomenological Analysis" (PhD diss., Saybrook University, 2015), accessed June 10, 2015, http://gradworks.umi.com/36/83/3683050.html.

18. A. L. Stanton et al., "Randomized, Controlled Trial of Written Emotional Expression and Benefit Finding in Breast Cancer Patients," *Journal of Clinical Oncology* 20, no. 20 (October 15, 2002: 4160–68.

19. Y. Sakai et al., "A Trial of Improvement of Immunity in Cancer Patients by Laughter Therapy," *Japan Hospitals* no. 32 (July 2013): 53–59.

CHAPTER 9: STRENGTHEN YOUR IMMUNE SYSTEM WITH SLEEP

1. "Sleepy Connected Americans: National Sleep Foundation Releases Annual Sleep in America Poll Exploring Connections with communications Technology Use

and Sleep," National Sleep Foundation, March 7, 2011, accessed January 25, 2015, http://sleepfoundation.org/media-center/press-release/annual-sleep-america-poll -exploring-connections-communications-technology-use.

2. University Hospitals Case Medical Center, "Lack of Sleep Found to Be a New Risk Factor for Aggressive Breast Cancers," *ScienceDaily*, accessed January 27, 2015, www.sciencedaily.com/releases/2012/08/120827113359.htm.

3. Lara G. Sigurdardóttir et al., "Sleep Disruption Among Older Men and Risk of Prostate Cancer," *Cancer Epidemiology, Biomarkers and Prevention* 22, no. 5 (May 2013): 872–79, doi: 10.1158/1055–9965.EPI-12–1227-T.

4. M. A. Martínez-Garcia et al., "Relationship Between Sleep Apnea and Cancer," *Archivos de bronconeumología Sociedad Española de Patología Respiratoria* (April 2, 2015), pii: S0300–2896(15)00074–5, doi: 10.1016/j.arbres.2015.02.002 [Epub ahead of print].

5. J. S. Chan et al., "Qigong Exercise Alleviates Fatigue, Anxiety, and Depressive Symptoms, Improves Sleep Quality, and Shortens Sleep Latency in Persons with Chronic Fatigue Syndrome-like Illness," *Evidence Based Complementary Alternative Medicine* (2014): 2014:106048, doi: 10.1155/2014/106048 [Epub December 25, 2014].

6. H. P. Landolt et al., "Late-Afternoon Ethanol Intake Affects Nocturnal Sleep and the Sleep EEG in Middle-aged Men," *Journal of Clinical Psychopharmacology* 16, no. 6 (1996): 428–36.

7. Joshua J. Gooley et al., "Exposure to Room Light Before Bedtime Suppresses Melatonin Onset and Shortens Melatonin Duration in Humans," *Journal of Clinical Endocrinology and Metabolism* 96, no. 3 (March 2011): E463–E472, doi: 10.1210/jc .2010–2098 PMCID: PMC3047226 [Epub December 30, 2010].

CHAPTER 11: CREATING AN ANTICANCER LIVING ENVIRONMENT

1. P. D. Darbre, F. Mannello, and C. Exley, "Aluminium and Breast Cancer: Sources of Exposure, Tissue Measurements and Mechanisms of Toxicological Actions on Breast Biology," *Journal of Inorganic Biochemistry* 128 (November 2013): 257–61. doi: 10.1016/j.jinorgbio.2013.07.005.

2. "Teflon Toxicosis Is Deadly to Pet Birds. Are We At Risk?" Environmental Working Group, (May 15, 2003), accessed February 18, 2015, http://www.ewg.org /research/canaries-kitchen.

3. Maria D. Guillen and Patricia S. Uriarte, "Aldehydes Contained in Edible Oils of a Very Different Nature After Prolonged Heating at Frying Temperature: Presence of Toxic Oxygenated A,B Unsaturated Aldehydes," *Food Chemistry*, 131, no. 3 (April 2012): 915–26.

4. Joe Mercola, "Why Did the Russians Ban an Appliance Found in 90% of Amer- ican Homes?" Mercola.com (May 18, 2010), accessed May 15, 2015, http://articles .mercola.com/sites/articles/archive/2010/05/18/microwave-hazards.aspx.

5. Lee Cowden and Connie Strasheim, *Create a Toxin-Free Body & Home Starting Today* (ACIM Press, 2014), 87–98.

6. Ritchie Shoemaker, *Mold Warriors* (Baltimore: Gateway Press, Inc., 2005); Ritchie Shoemaker, "Policy Holders of America: Research Committee Report on Diagnosis and Treatment of Chronic Inflammatory Response Syndrome Caused by Exposure to the Interior Environment of Water-Damaged Buildings," SurvivingMold. com, accessed February 18, 2015, SurvivingMold.com/legal-resources/publications /poa-position-statement-paper.

CHAPTER 14: LIVING A CANCER-FREE LIFE

1. Preetha Anand et al., "Cancer Is a Preventable Disease That Requires Major Lifestyle Changes," *Pharmaceutical Research* 25, no. 9 (September 2008): 2097–2116, doi: 10.1007/s11095–008–9661–9 [Epub July 15, 2008].

Recipe List

Fresh Blender Juices

Spicy Green
Ginger Snap
Simply Greens Detox Beverage
Sweet Greens
Fresh Veggie Juice

Protein Powder Veggie Juice
Fresh Gazpacho Blender Juice
Ginger Lemon Drink
Mega Greens Drink
Apple Drink

Nut Milks and Protein Powder Drinks

Basic Homemade Nut Milk
Mocha Nut Milk Shake

Coco Loco Nut Shake
Whey or Plant Protein Powder Drink

Basic Beverages

Lemon/Limeade
Iced Green Tea
Anti-Inflammatory Tea

Fiber Drink
Cider Vinegar Drink
Savory Sipping Alkaline Broth

Fast and Easy Breakfasts

Poached Eggs
Hard-Boiled Eggs
Turkey Bacon

Dips, Sauces, and Marinades

Fresh Mayonnaise

MCT Metabolically
    Friendly Mayonnaise

Spicy Burger Sauce

Fresh Salsa

Fresh Guacamole

Tomato and Basil Topping

Parsley Pesto

Pine Nut or Walnut Dip

Curry Sauce

Creamy Curry Dip

Dijon Chicken Marinade

Lamb or Beef Marinade

Italian Marinade

Teriyaki Marinade

Asian Marinade

Ginger Citrus Marinade

Salads and Salad Dressings

Dressings

MCT Essential Salad Dressing

French Salad Dressing

Citrus Delight Dressing

Cilantro Salad Dressing

Basil Salad Dressing

Creamy Garlic Dressing

Caesar Salad Dressing

Hearty Salads

Baby Greens Side Salad

Arugula Side Salad

Kale Side Salad

Greek Side Salad

Nutty Greek Salad

Greek Salad with Chicken

Chinese Chicken Salad

Curry Chicken Salad

Chicken Caesar Salad

Ceviche Salad

Seared Toasted Sesame Salmon Salad

Salmon Salad with Avocado

Sautéed Scallops Seafood Salad

Filling Soups

Miso Broth with Mushrooms

Vegetable Soup

Vegetable Medley Soup

Creamy Broccoli/Cauliflower Soup

Chicken Vegetable Soup

Hearty Beef Soup

Seafood and Coconut Milk Soup with Cilantro and Chives

Side Dishes
Steamed Artichokes
Steamed Cauliflower Delight
Fennel with Turmeric
Steamed Dill Carrots
Roasted Zucchini and Eggplant

Easy Entrées
Zucchini Noodles
Baby Rack of Lamb
Filet Mignon
Dijon Dill Salmon
Tex-Mex Turkey Wraps
Herb Almond Crusted Chicken or Mahimahi
Garlic Lemon Dijon Chicken
Chili Beef Wraps
Ground Chicken or Turkey Patties (with Lettuce Wrap)
Versatile Meat Loaf
Garlic Herbed Shrimp

Simple Snacks and Desserts
Crunchy Seed Snack Mix
Sprouted Nuts
Toasted Nuts
Cheesy Cashew Kale Chips
Deviled Eggs
Raw Low-Carbohydrate Chocolate Squares
Cinnamon Chia Pudding

Acknowledgments

Love is the medicine and solution for everything.

I am so blessed and thankful for my husband, Patrick, who lets me explore all the possibilities of the universe and be a free spirit. I am also blessed for my wonderful children, Brittany, Brooke, Robert, Breanne, Beth, Alannah, and Grant, who constantly inspire me.

In addition, I am thankful for all of the people in my life who have contributed to my growth and development: my parents, teachers, and therapists, as well as my beautiful, dear friends, whose love and friendship are priceless.

I am thankful for those who have taught me about integrative and new medicine, especially Lee Cowden, MD, who has pushed me to rise to the occasion to educate and train other doctors.

I am also thankful for all the following people:

Jonathan Wright, MD, who masterfully educates many practitioners on well-researched protocols for everyday medical problems.

Bill Coury, who was a cancer survivor who illuminated my path to care for cancer patients.

Deepok Chopra, who first taught me how to meditate and initiated my understanding about Ayurvedic medicine.

Sherry Rogers, MD, who has dedicated her entire being to writing books about everything in medicine and who very carefully references all of her work.

Garry Gordon, MD, who inspires and informs anybody who will listen about what to do to have the most optimal, outstanding health.

Burton Goldberg, who is as old as the Queen of England and who never ceases to share everything that he knows about integrative medicine all over the world.

I also want to acknowledge those who are involved in organizations, such as the American College for Advancement in Medicine (ACAM) and the Academy for Comprehensive Integrative Medicine (ACIM), whose leadership and members devote their energy and time to educating practitioners on the latest and greatest discoveries of new medicine.

I give thanks for my amazing team of doctors, health practitioners, and the rest of my staff, who diligently work daily to help and support this great movement. These include Liliana Partida, our illustrious nutritionist, whose understanding in the science of food and nutrition contributed to our recipes throughout the book.

My deepest appreciation also goes to Connie Strasheim, for her brilliance as a writer in helping me to create this book, and for her love and devotion to bring great understanding to a complex topic.

Last but not least, I want to thank my patients, who have been a part of my evolving journey and who teach me much, just as I teach them, and are willing to be adventurous in their healing journey.

General Index

Recipe Index

Leigh Erin Connealy, MD

LEIGH ERIN CONNEALY, MD, has been practicing medicine for thirty years, since 1986. She is founder and medical director of the Center for New Medicine and the Cancer Center for Healing in Irvine, California, which provide cutting-edge treatments for cancer and other chronic, degenerative diseases. Dr. Connealy and her staff go beyond the limitations of conventional medicine and heal the root causes of disease using state-of-the-art, science-based whole-body medicine, compassion, and love. She believes in treating the patient with the disease, not the disease of the patient.

Dr. Connealy educates other health professionals and her lectures and articles have been published in multiple scientific publications. In her newsletter, Newport Natural Health, she daily shares free tools for improving health with natural medicine. She has appeared on numerous television programs and for ten years was a weekly cohost on Frank Jordan's national radio show Healthy, Wealthy and Wise.

Dr. Connealy is founder of Perfectly Healthy, a company that provides supplements that contain all of the vitamins, minerals, and nutrients that are missing from the Standard American Diet (SAD). These are available through the Perfectly Healthy online store maintained by Dr. Connealy and the Center for New Medicine.

To learn more about Leigh Erin Connealy, MD, or the Cancer Center for Healing, see www.connealymd.com and www.cancercenterforhealingcom.